D1263888

CARBOHYDRATE BIOCHEMISTRY AND METABOLISM

Related AVI Books

CARBOHYDRATE BIOCHEMISTRY AND METABOLISM

Karla L. Roehrig
Department of Food Science
and Nutrition
The Ohio State University
Columbus, Ohio

AVI PUBLISHING COMPANY, INC.
Westport, Connecticut

Library of Congress Cataloging in Publication Data

Roehrig, Karla L.
  Carbohydrate biochemistry and metabolism.

  Includes bibliographies and index.
  1. Carbohydrates—Metabolism.   2. Carbohydrates—
Metabolism—Disorders.   I. Title.
QP701.R58   1984   599'.01'33   83-22476
ISBN 0-87055-447-6

Printed in the United States of America

To my husband and my parents

Contents

Preface

This book is the result of an advanced graduate course on carbohydrates at The Ohio State University, and I would especially like to thank the members of the spring 1981 class for their questions and comments, which aided in selection of topics to be included in this text.

This text is intended for use by advanced undergraduate and graduate students wishing to know more about the biochemistry and metabolism of various classes of carbohydrates. It presupposes a knowledge of organic chemistry and general biochemistry. It is hoped it will also serve as a useful reference text for researchers whose area of expertise may not be carbohydrate biochemistry but who may have a need for knowledge of the various carbohydrate pathways and their regulation.

An attempt has been made to encompass the carbohydrate biochemistry and metabolism of higher animals, distinguishing where necessary between ruminants and nonruminants. Some sections will, of course, be slanted more toward one species or another. Part I of the book provides a brief review of carbohydrate chemistry, while the last section reviews several of the numerous industrial uses for carbohydrates.

I am deeply indebted to my colleagues, Drs. T. Kristoffersen, J. Allred, and J. Goodson, for their advice, encouragement, and support during the preparation of this manuscript. For any errors of omission or commission, however, I accept the sole responsibility. Ms. B. Bezouska deserves considerable appreciation for her patient and careful translation of my handwriting into typescript. I particularly wish to thank my husband, Dr. Fred Roehrig, for his patience and encouragement throughout this endeavor.

Karla L. Roehrig

Introduction

The largest amount of any single biochemical compound on Earth is a carbohydrate, cellulose. Chitin, the carbohydrate found in insect and crustacean cytoskeletans, also contributes a large percentage to the total biomass. Carbohydrates comprise a significant proportion of the stored nutrients in both plant (starch) and animal (glycogen) cells and also serve as much of the short-term energy supply (glucose) of cells. In addition to serving as nutrients, they make up a good deal of the structural material of the cell: cellulose and hemicellulose in plants, chitin in insects, and crustaceans and hyaluronic acid and chondroitin sulfate in higher animals. Carbohydrates are also involved in the processes by which cells recognize each other. In addition to serving directly, carbohydrates are metabolized to yield many of the other building blocks of the cell. They also have many industrial uses as well, such as for gels and thickeners and, of course, for alcohol production.

In light of the important role of carbohydrates in the biochemical function of plants and animals, it is important that we understand and appreciate the chemistry, biochemistry, and metabolism of these compounds. To date, the study of carbohydrate metabolism (notably glycogen metabolism) has provided a great deal of information about the regulatory processes in the cell. Many of the diseases of man and animals are related to a malfunction in carbohydrate metabolism.

The purpose of this book is to provide a review of carbohydrate chemistry, biochemistry, and metabolism and to develop an appreciation for the regulation of the various pathways in carbohydrate metabolism. This approach to carbohydrate metabolism, it is hoped, will provide the reader with the tools and information to understand the anomalies of carbohydrate metabolism in man and animals.

Each part covers some significant aspect of the chemistry, biochemistry, metabolism, or applied use of carbohydrates. Within each part are several chapters dealing with these topics. At the end of each chapter are some general references to provide a basis for further reading. Where possible, these will be review articles or books. Additionally, there will be specific references cited in the text. Together, this bibliography, while certainly not intended to be comprehensive, will aid the student to delve more deeply into each area. Each chapter will also have a few review questions at the end designed to test the reader's comprehension of the material in that chapter.

Part I

Carbohydrate Chemistry and Nomenclature

Carbohydrate Monomers

A. HISTORICAL BACKGROUND

Initially, the name carbohydrate was assigned to sugars and their polymers because it was thought that they followed the general formula $C_n(H_2O)_n$. Now, however, these componds are more properly described as *polyhydroxy*aldehydes, ketones, alcohols, acids, amines, or their condensation products.

Although the presence of a sweet substance in urine from diabetics was noted in an ancient Egyptian papyrus, and grape sugar was discussed in twelfth century Moorish writing, it was not until 1747 that Andreas Marggraf isolated sucrose from sugar beets and showed that the sugar (glucose) from raisins was distinct. In 1811, Kerchoff demonstrated that acid hydrolysis of starch led to the formation of a syrup containing an isolatable sugar. In 1838 Dumas named the sugar found after starch hydrolysis (as well as in urine from diabetics and in grapes) glucose. It was the work of Emil Fischer, however, that led to the elucidation of the structure of glucose and a number of other carbohydrates in the early 1900s. He outlined a number of steps that aided in determining structure. Ultimately C. S. Hudson formally put these steps together into what is now commonly referred to as Fischer's proof. It was known that there were different isomers with differing chemical properties but with the same empirical formula and that the same osazone was derived from glucose, mannose, and fructose. When glucose and mannose were oxidized by hot nitric acid, optically active aldaric acids resulted. When the pentose arabinose was subjected to the Kiliani cyanohydrin synthesis enantiomers of the aldonic acids prepared from glucose and mannose were the result. By comparing which pairs of enantiomers could give rise to such compounds, the configuration of glucose was deduced. It was only much later that X-ray crystallography was used to prove that the arbitrarily assigned D and L configurations were correct in an absolute sense.

After the structural determinations of various carbohydrates were made, interest in carbohydrate research declined. This was due in part to difficulties inherent in this field of study. Complex carbohydrates especially pose difficulties because they are multifunctional with many potential reactive sites. Sequencing of the polysaccharides does not enjoy the aid of techniques that exist for sequencing proteins or nucleic acids. It is also troublesome to synthesize artificial carbohydrates of known sequence. Naturally occurring carbohydrates are branched compounds whereas the study of proteins and nucleic acids is facilitated because these are linear molecules. All of these structural properties have served as barriers to carbohydrate research.

B. MONOSACCHARIDES

Carbohydrates may be classified as *mono-, di-, tri-, oligo-,* or *poly-saccharides* depending on whether they are made of one, two, three, two–ten, or more than ten monomeric units, respectively. The *mono-saccharides* are referred to as "simple sugars." Although there are more than 200 known monosaccharides, D-glucose is the most abundant in nature. D-Glucose is an *aldose* or *aldosugar* because it has a carbonyl group at the end of the carbon chain making it an aldehyde. Other sugars may be aldosugars as well. If, however, the carbonyl is at any position other than the terminal position, then the sugars are *ketoses* or *ketosugars*.

In this book we will be concerned chiefly with the D series of sugars; by convention this includes all those saccharides where the hydroxyl on the asymmetric carbon farthest away from the carbonyl group is on the right. L-Glucose is the mirror image of D-glucose (Fig. 1.1). The asymmetric carbons and the convention for numbering carbons are shown. Since there are four asymmetric carbons there are 16 possible *isomers* of the six carbon aldoses (hexoses). Eight of these are D sugars and eight are L sugars. Initially, the D configuration was arbitrarily assigned to dextrorotatory glyceraldehyde, and thus, to all compounds with the same relative orientation as D-glyceraldehyde. Now it is known that the absolute configuration of D-glyceraldehyde is correct.

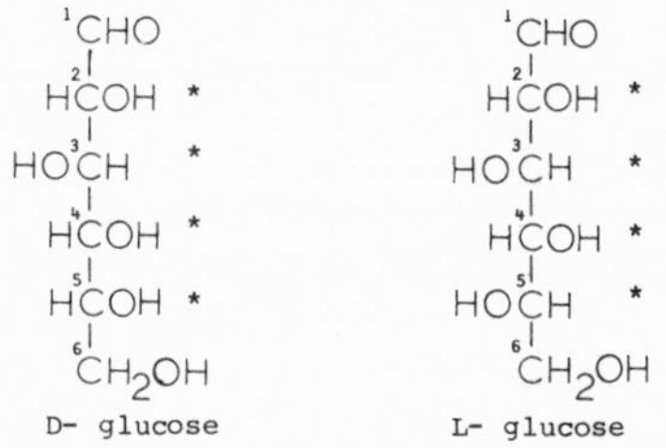

$$^1CHO$$
$$^2HCOH \quad *$$
$$HO^3CH \quad *$$
$$^4HCOH \quad *$$
$$^5HCOH \quad *$$
$$^6CH_2OH$$
D- glucose

$$^1CHO$$
$$^2HCOH \quad *$$
$$HO^3CH \quad *$$
$$^4HCOH \quad *$$
$$HO^5CH \quad *$$
$$^6CH_2OH$$
L- glucose

FIG. 1.1. The structures of D- and L-glucose.

The simplest D-aldosugar is glyceraldehyde. Its four (aldotetrose), five (aldopentose), and six (aldohexose) carbon relatives are shown in Fig. 1.2. It is relatively easy to remember the structures of these compounds: one may rely not on memory but on a mnemonic trick. D-Gly-

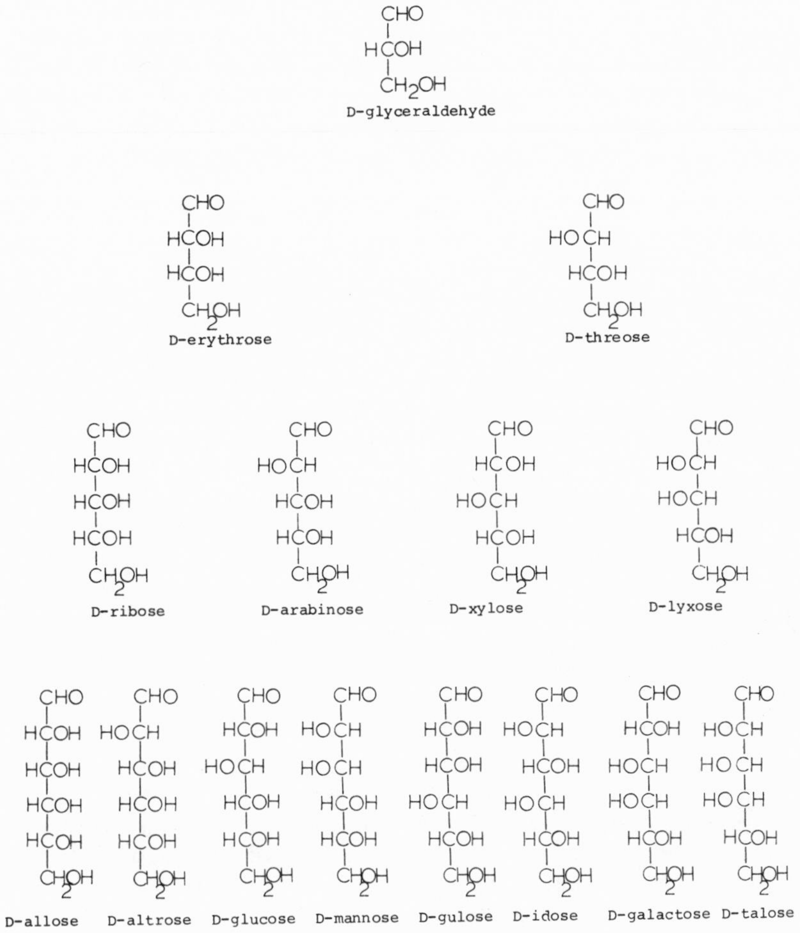

CHO
|
HCOH
|
CH₂OH
D-glyceraldehyde

CHO
|
HCOH
|
HCOH
|
CH₂OH
D-erythrose

CHO
|
HOCH
|
HCOH
|
CH₂OH
D-threose

CHO
|
HCOH
|
HCOH
|
HCOH
|
CH₂OH
D-ribose

CHO
|
HOCH
|
HCOH
|
HCOH
|
CH₂OH
D-arabinose

CHO
|
HCOH
|
HOCH
|
HCOH
|
CH₂OH
D-xylose

CHO
|
HOCH
|
HOCH
|
HCOH
|
CH₂OH
D-lyxose

CHO
|
HCOH
|
HCOH
|
HCOH
|
HCOH
|
CH₂OH
D-allose

CHO
|
HOCH
|
HCOH
|
HCOH
|
HCOH
|
CH₂OH
D-altrose

CHO
|
HCOH
|
HOCH
|
HCOH
|
HCOH
|
CH₂OH
D-glucose

CHO
|
HOCH
|
HOCH
|
HCOH
|
HCOH
|
CH₂OH
D-mannose

CHO
|
HCOH
|
HCOH
|
HOCH
|
HCOH
|
CH₂OH
D-gulose

CHO
|
HOCH
|
HCOH
|
HOCH
|
HCOH
|
CH₂OH
D-idose

CHO
|
HCOH
|
HOCH
|
HOCH
|
HCOH
|
CH₂OH
D-galactose

CHO
|
HOCH
|
HOCH
|
HOCH
|
HCOH
|
CH₂OH
D-talose

FIG. 1.2.   The D series of aldose monosaccharides.

ceraldehyde has only one possible structure since it has only one asymmetric carbon. There is, of course, another isomer, but it is the L isomer. For the aldotetroses there are 2^2 or 4 isomers two of which are D forms. These are erythrose and threose. The aldopentoses have four D forms: ribose, arabinose, xylose, and lyxose. To determine the positions of the hydroxyls, draw four five-carbon chains (Fig. 1.3). Put the aldehyde groups on all the top carbons, the H_2OH on the bottom carbons, and a hydroxyl to the right on the next to the bottom (fourth) carbons. Now divide the pentoses into two equal groups (2 and 2). Starting on the left side of the page put hydroxyls on the right of carbon three for the first group and on the left for the second group. Divide each group

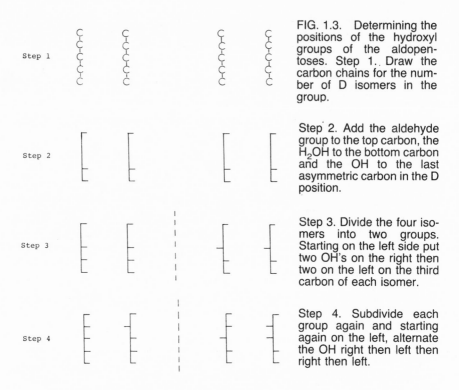

Step 1

Step 2

Step 3

Step 4

FIG. 1.3. Determining the positions of the hydroxyl groups of the aldopentoses. Step 1. Draw the carbon chains for the number of D isomers in the group.

Step 2. Add the aldehyde group to the top carbon, the H_2OH to the bottom carbon and the OH to the last asymmetric carbon in the D position.

Step 3. Divide the four isomers into two groups. Starting on the left side put two OH's on the right then two on the left on the third carbon of each isomer.

Step 4. Subdivide each group again and starting again on the left, alternate the OH right then left then right then left.

in half again, and alternate the hydroxyls right, left, right, left. The acronym for this group is RAXL, so starting from the left name the isomers ribose, arabinose, xylose, and lyxose. The same procedure is used for the aldohexoses; there is just one more subgroup involved. To aid in remembering the names of the aldohexoses the phrase *all altrose gladly make gum in gallon tanks* or allose, altrose, glucose, mannose, gulose, idose, galactose, and talose is useful.

The ketose series is shown in Fig. 1.4. Dihydroxyacetone has only one isomer because it has no asymmetric carbons. There are two (2^1) four carbon, four (2^2) five carbon, and eight (2^3) six carbon ketoses, only half of which are D-ketoses. The process by which one can remember the positioning of the hydroxyl groups is similar to the aldohexose group. Draw the carbon chain, then put an H_2OH on C-1, a carbonyl on C-2, a hydroxyl to the right on the last asymmetric carbon, and an H_2OH on the last carbon. Proceed to divide the sugars into subgroups and distribute the hydroxyls as demonstrated for the aldohexoses. Sugars that differ from each other only in the configuration about one carbon are *epimers*.

In solution, sugars often behave as if there is one more asymmetric carbon than the structures would indicate. For example, when pure D-glucose is in solution, there appear to be two isomers (named α and

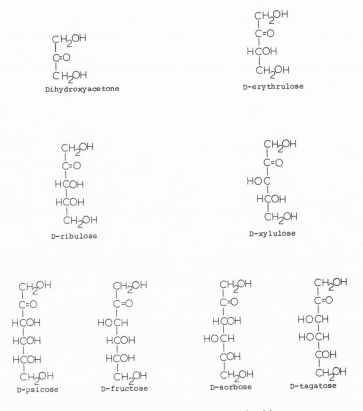

FIG. 1.4.　The D series of ketose monosaccharides.

β) with differing physical properties. An equilibrium mixture of these two isomers consists of ⅓α and ⅔β. Glucose oxidase can metabolize the β form 100% and the α form less than 1%. The melting points are different: α = 146°C vs. β = 150°C. The α form is less soluble in water (82.5 g/100 ml) than the β form (178 g/100 ml). This additional asymmetry arises because instead of being linear compounds in solution, such sugars form *heterocyclic rings*, rings composed of more than one type of atom. D-Glucose forms a pyran-type ring (a five carbon heterocyclic ring and is therefore called D-glucopyranose. The α and β forms are shown in ring form in Fig. 1.5. The ring results because of a general type of reaction between an aldehyde and an alcohol to form a *hemiacetal*. D-Glucopyranose is therefore an *internal hemiacetal* where the C-5 hydroxyl has reacted with the C-1 aldehyde. Isomeric forms that differ in configuration only around the carbonyl carbon are called *anomers*. Thus, the carbonyl carbon is the *anomeric carbon*. All aldoses with at least five carbons can form stable pyranose rings.

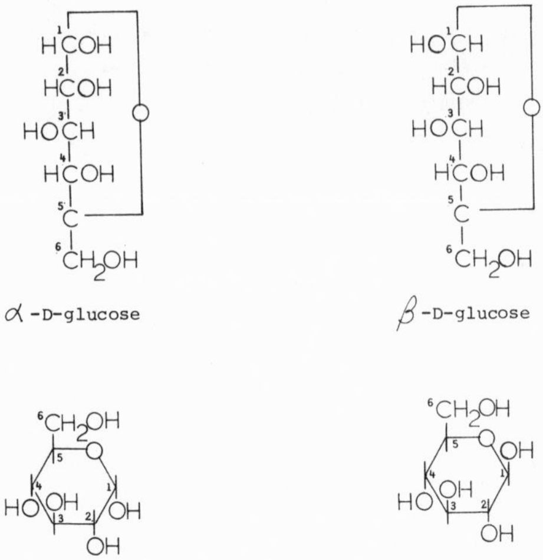

$$
\begin{array}{ll}
H^1COH & HO^1CH \\
H^2COH & H^2COH \\
HO^3CH & HO^3CH \\
H^4COH & H^4COH \\
^5C & ^5C \\
^6CH_2OH & ^6CH_2OH
\end{array}
$$

α -D-glucose β -D-glucose

FIG. 1.5. The heterocyclic (top and conventional (bottom) ring structures of α- and β-D-glucose.

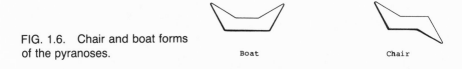

C. AXIAL AND EQUITORIAL CONFIGURATIONS

The ring structures are not really planar as shown in Fig. 1.5 but instead form strained rings called either boat or chair forms (Fig. 1.6). The chair form is more rigid and more stable than the boat form. The

FIG. 1.6. Chair and boat forms of the pyranoses.

Boat   Chair

substituent groups are neither chemically nor geometrically equivalent. They may be *axial,* parallel to the axis of symmetry, or *equitorial,* perpendicular to the axis of symmetry (Fig. 1-7). Equitorial groups are more readily esterified than are axial groups.

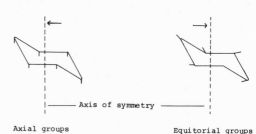

——— Axis of symmetry ———

FIG. 1.7. Axial and equitorial positions on the chair form.   Axial groups   Equitorial groups

The chair form itself has two conformations called C-1 and 1-C (Fig. 1.8). Most D-pyranoses are in the C-1 conformation. The conformation that a sugar preferentially takes, however, depends on the maximization of the equitorial groups. In general, the most stable conformation is the one in which the CH_2OH group is equitorial, but if several equitorial hydroxyl groups could be obtained by allowing the existence of an axial CH_2OH group, then the 1-C position is the preferred one.

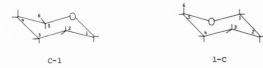

FIG. 1.8. Distribution of axial and equitorial bonds in the C-1 and 1-C conformations.

Such is the case with D-idose, which gains 4 equitorial hydroxyl groups by allowing the CH_2OH to assume the axial position. It is not surprising that β-D-glucopyranose is the most stable, most abundant sugar since in the C-1 conformation, all of its bulky groups can assume equitorial positions (Fig. 1.9); α-D-glucose is a less preferred sugar since the anomeric hydroxyl group would of necessity be axial.

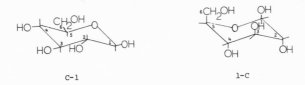

FIG. 1.9. The C-1 and 1-C conformations of β-D- glucopyranose.

It is a rather easy matter to determine whether bonds are axial or equitorial. First, draw the C-1 and 1-C chair forms with the oxygens in the ring. Start around the ring clockwise from the oxygen, remembering that the first axial bond will be as far away from the oxygen as possible. So if the oxygen is up (C-1), then the first axial will be down, the next up, the third down, the fourth up, and the fifth down. If the oxygen is down (1-C), then the first axial will be up, the second down, and so on. The equitorial positions are then easily added. To actually place the hydroxyl groups, remember that substituents to the right in a linear structure are always down on a ring. Further, for D-sugars the CH_2OH must always be in the up position regardless of whether that position is axial or equitorial. The two conformations of D-mannose are illustrated in Fig. 1.10. It is clear that the C-1 β-D-mannose is the preferred configuration because there are 4 equitorial substituents and 1 axial substituent in this conformation.

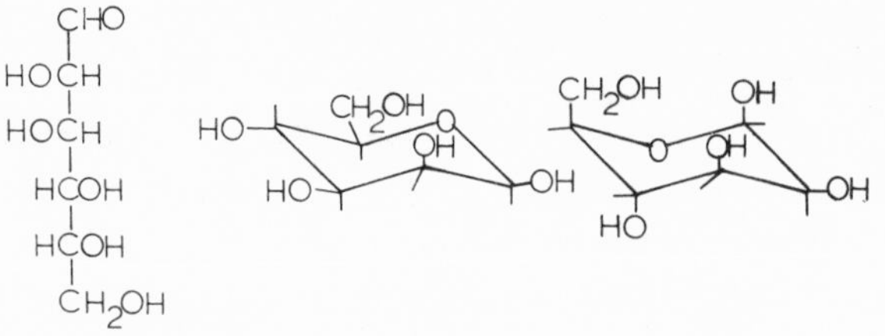

D-mannose

C-1
4 equitorial
1 axial

1-C
1 equitorial
4 axial

FIG. 1.10.   Conformations of β-D-mannose.

Five or six membered ketoses may form a furanose ring in solution. This occurs as the result of the condensation of a ketone and alcohol to form a *hemiketal*. The ring structure of β-D-fructose is commonly shown as the furanose form (Fig. 1.11). Prince *et al.* (1982) have shown that the predominant form of fructose is actually a pyranose and that at room temperature fructose is distributed 67% β-D-fructopyranose, 27% β-D-fructofuranose, 6% α-D-fructofuranose, and a trace of the open chain form. Although aldohexoses can exist in furanose ring forms the pyranose ring is more stable and predominates in solution.

FIG. 1.11.   Structure of
β-D-fructofuranose.

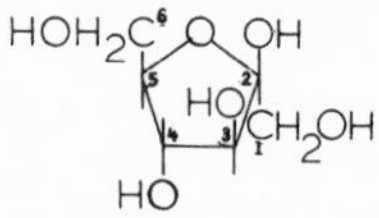

D. REACTIONS OF MONOSACCHARIDES

It is possible to determine whether a sugar is a pyranose or furanose by treating it with periodic acid, which cleaves adjacent hydroxyl groups. A furanose will yield a dialdehyde whereas a pyranose will yield a dialdehyde and formic acid (Fig. 1.12).

It is also possible to determine whether a sugar is a *reducing sugar*, that is, whether it has a free anomeric carbon and thus is capable of reducing Fehling's reagent (an alkaline copper tartrate complex), Benedict's solution (an alkaline copper citrate solution), or Tollen's reagent [$AG(NH_3)_2 \rightarrow Ag^0$].

Carbohydrates may undergo a number of general reactions, either chemically or enzymatically. Among these reactions are *reductions, oxidations, rearrangements, dehydrations, addition reactions, glycoside formation, condensation,* and *reactions of the alcohol groups.* An example of each type is shown in Table 1.1. All of the reactions shown are enzymatic but corresponding chemical reactions are also known for each group.

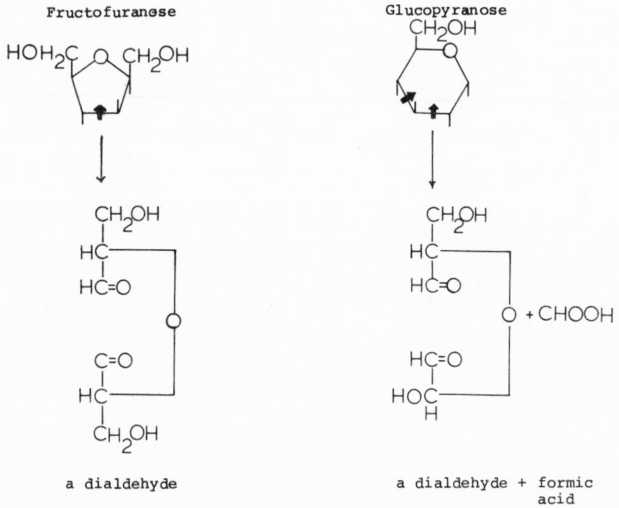

FIG. 1.12. Periodic acid cleavage of furanoses and pyranoses.

TABLE 1.1. Possible Reactions of Carbohydrates

Reaction type	Example	Enzyme
Reduction	Ribulose-5-P → Ribitol-5-P	Ribitol-phosphate dehydrogenase
Oxidation	Glucose-6-P → 6-P-gluconolactone	Glucose-6-P dehydrogenase
Rearrangement	Glyceraldehyde-3-P → DHAP	Triose-phosphate isomerase
Dehydration	2-glycerophosphate → PEP	Enolase
Additions	Arabinose + nitromethane → glucose + mannose	Sowden–Fischer synthesis
Glycoside formation	UDPglucose + glycogen$_n$ → glycogen^{n+1}	Glycogen synthetase
Condensation	Glyceraldehyde-3-P + DHAP → fructose 1,6-bisphosphate	Aldolase
Alcohol group reactions	GDPmannose → GDP 4-keto-6-deoxymannose	GDPmannose 4-oxido-6-reductase

E. SUMMARY

Carbohydrates are classified according to the number of monomeric units they possess. The monomers that make up carbohydrates may be aldo- or ketosugars depending on the location of the carbonyl carbon. A number of isomers may be possible depending on the number of asymmetric carbons present. These isomers have differing physical and chemical properties. Monomers of five or more carbons frequently form heterocyclic rings, which lead to an apparent extra asymmetric carbon called the anomeric carbon. The rings themselves can assume several spatial orientations, the most likely of which being the one with a minimum amount of strain energy (maximized equitorial bonds). The study of complex carbohydrates has been hindered because of their structural characteristics: they have many reactive sites and are often highly branched.

REVIEW QUESTIONS

1. Define
    a. Anomers
    b. Epimers
    c. Furanose
    d. Pyranose
    e. Isomers
2. What is the 2-epimer of D-glucose?
3. How many axial and equitorial substituents does β-D-allose have in the C-1 and 1-C conformations?
4. Periodic acid treatment of a sugar yielded a dialdehyde and formic acid. Was it a pyranose or a furanose?

BIBLIOGRAPHY

Barker, R. 1971. Organic Chemistry of Biological Compounds. Prentice-Hall, Inc., Englewood Cliffs, New Jersey.
Lehninger, A. 1975. Biochemistry, 2nd Edition. Worth Publishers, New York.
Morrison, R., and Boyd, R. 1976. Organic Chemistry, 3rd Edition. Allyn and Bacon, Boston, Massachusetts.
Prince, R., Gunson, D., Leigh, J., and McDonald, G. 1982. The predominant form of fructose is a pyranose, not a furanose ring. Trends Biochem. Sci. 7, 239–240.
Sharon, N. 1980. Carbohydrates. Sci. Am. November, p. 90.

2

Types of Simple Carbohydrates

A. AMINO SUGARS AND OTHER DERIVATIVES

The monosaccharides are not restricted to having merely hydroxyl groups as substituents. There are a number of physiologically important amine sugars, e.g., glucosamine, galactosamine, and nucleic acids such as cytidine (Fig. 2.1).* Glucosamine is a major component of

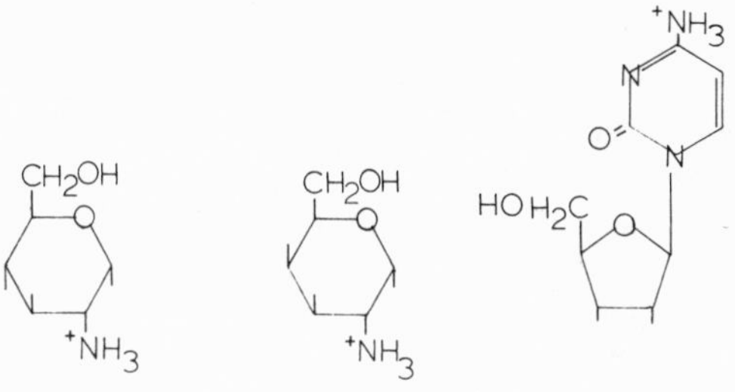

α-D-glucosamine α-D-galactosamine   N(β-D-ribofuranosyl) cytosine

FIG. 2.1.   Some physiologically important amino sugars.

chitin and galactosamine is found in abundance in the cartilage polysaccharide chondroitin sulfate. There are also O-methyl derivatives (Fig. 2.2). In addition, sugars also undergo reduction of the carbonyl group to an alcohol forming sugar alcohols such as mannitol, xylitol, and glycerol (Fig. 2.3). N-Acetyl groups may be substituents yielding such compounds as N-acetylglucosamine.

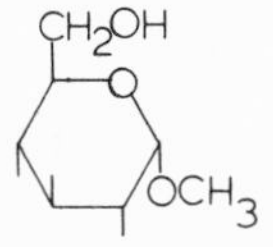

FIG. 2.2.   An O-methyl derivative of glucose.

methyl-α-D-glucopyranoside

*From this point on, hydroxyl groups will be denoted by a line perpendicular to the plain of the ring.

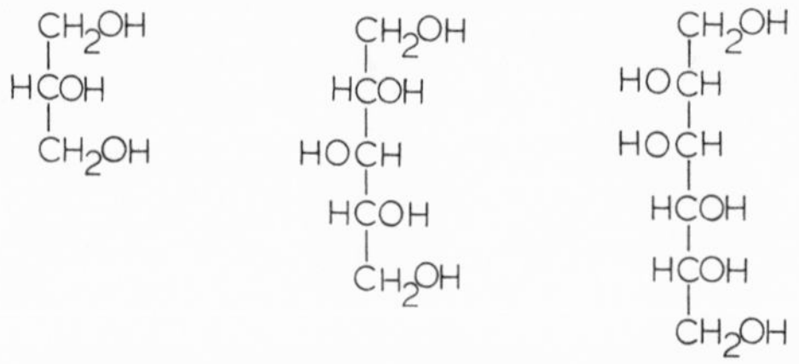

$$
\begin{array}{ccc}
\text{CH}_2\text{OH} & \text{CH}_2\text{OH} & \text{CH}_2\text{OH} \\
| & | & | \\
\text{HCOH} & \text{HCOH} & \text{HOCH} \\
| & | & | \\
\text{CH}_2\text{OH} & \text{HOCH} & \text{HOCH} \\
 & | & | \\
 & \text{HCOH} & \text{HCOH} \\
 & | & | \\
 & \text{CH}_2\text{OH} & \text{HCOH} \\
 & & | \\
 & & \text{CH}_2\text{OH} \\
\text{Glycerol} & \text{Xylitol} & \text{Mannitol}
\end{array}
$$

FIG. 2.3. Sugar alcohols.

B. SUGAR ACIDS

The sugar acids form an important class. These are made by oxidation to form a carboxylic acid. There are three possible types of sugar acids: *aldonic, aldaric,* and *uronic* acids (Fig. 2.4). Aldonic acids are formed when only the aldehyde carbon is oxidized which results in a compound typified by gluconic acid. The aldaric acids are formed as the result of oxidation of both the aldehyde carbon and the C-6 carbon. D-Glucaric acid is an example of this group. Although the aldaric acids are useful experimentally, they serve little biological purpose. The uronic acids, on the other hand, are very important biologically. They exist as the result of the oxidation of the number 6 carbon resulting in such compounds as glucuronic, galacturonic, and mannuronic acids. The uronic acids are important in the detoxification of many drugs and biological products and are also constituents of many polysaccharides. They may also form lactones. One sugar acid of considerable importance is ascorbic acid (vitamin C). The phosphorylated forms of sugar acids play a crucial role in metabolism and are represented by such compounds as glucose 1-phosphate, fructose 6-phosphate, fructose 1,6-bisphosphate, and glyceraldehyde 3-phosphate.

$$
\begin{array}{ccc}
\text{Aldonic} & \text{Aldaric} & \text{Uronic} \\
\text{COOH} & \text{COOH} & \text{CHO} \\
| & | & | \\
\text{COH} & \text{HCOH} & \text{HCOH} \\
| & | & | \\
\text{HOC} & \text{HOCH} & \text{HOCH} \\
| & | & | \\
\text{HCOH} & \text{HCOH} & \text{HCOH} \\
| & | & | \\
\text{HCOH} & \text{HCOH} & \text{HCOH} \\
| & | & | \\
\text{CH}_2\text{OH} & \text{COOH} & \text{COOH} \\
\text{D-gluconic acid} & \text{D-glucaric acid} & \text{D-glucuronic acid}
\end{array}
$$

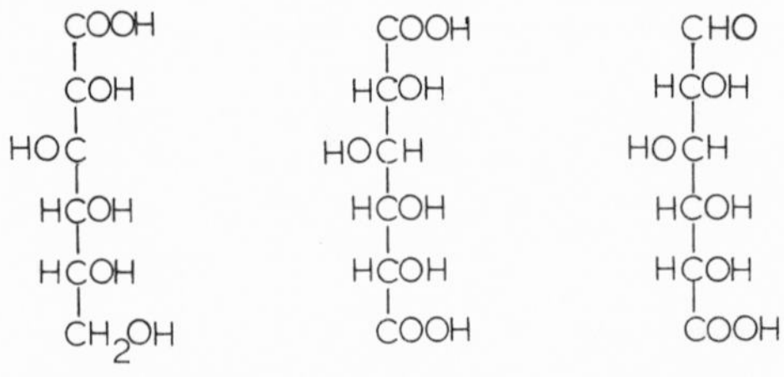

FIG. 2.4. Sugar acids.

C. DEOXYSUGARS

Deoxysugars form another important category. The most abundant of these sugars is 2-deoxyribose (Fig. 2.5), which is the sugar moiety of

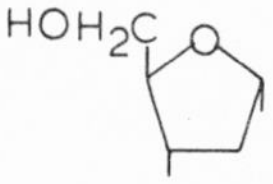

FIG. 2.5.   Deoxysugars.   2-deoxyribose

DNA. Rhamnose (6-deoxymannose) and fucose (6-deoxygalactose) are important components of bacterial cell walls, in the form of lipopolysaccharides. It is the polymers of these and similar sugars which give the cell walls high tensile strength.

D. MURAMIC AND NEURAMINIC ACIDS

There are some other important monomers such as muramic acid and neuraminic acid found in bacterial cell walls and the cell coats of higher animals, respectively (Fig. 2.6). The N-acetyl derivative of neuramic acid is sialic acid, which is the form found most often in humans. Sialic acid is extremely important in the half-life timing of plasma proteins and also in cell–cell recognition. In other species there is a high content of the N-glycoyl derivative. In bacterial cells, the cell wall is extremely important to cellular integrity. Whereas mammalian cells are surrounded by the comfort of an isotonic media, bacterial cells may be faced with hostile environments of low or high ionic strengths. Bacteria fall roughly into two classes depending on the amount of lipid in their cell walls which determines their reaction with Gram stain. Gram-positive cells have little lipid while gram-negative cells are lipid rich. Both categories, however, have tough, resilient polysaccharide–protein complexes comprising the cell wall. This complex is called *murein* and is composed of a *muropeptide* repeating unit. A fundamental muropeptide is N-acetyl glucosamine $\beta(1 \rightarrow 4)$-N-acetylmuramic

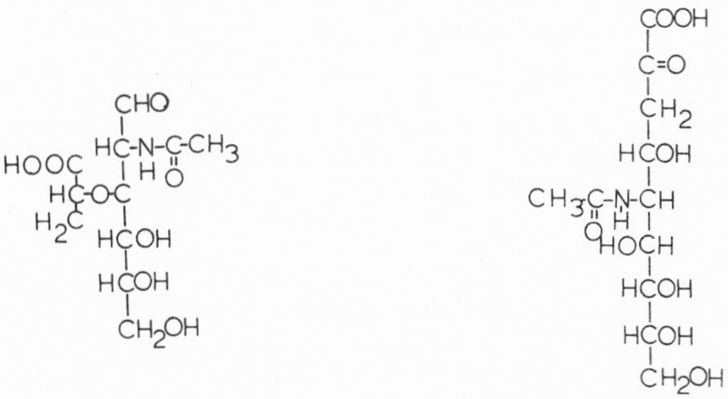

Muramic acid

N-acetyl neuraminic
acid (sialic acid)

FIG. 2.6.   Muramic and N-acetylneuraminic acids.

acid with a tetrapeptide of L-alanine, D-glutamate, L-lysine, and D-alanine covalently linked to the lactic acid moiety of muramic acid. Cross-linking between amino acid side chains by amino acid bridges causes the polymer to form a netlike matrix. Lysozyme, an enzyme that causes rupture of gram-positive bacteria, is a hydrolase that attacks the β(1 → 4) glycosidic linkages between the carbohydrates. In addition to the murein matrix other polymers strengthen the cell walls. These include teichoic acids, which are chains of glycerol or ribitol, polymers of rhamnose, glucose, mannose, or galactose and their derivatives, and polypeptides. Gram-negative cells also contain lipopolysaccharides. Final assembly of these components occurs on the outside of the cell walls.

E. DISACCHARIDES

Disaccharides are composed of two monosaccharides connected by a glycosidic linkage. Some of the more common disaccharides are maltose, lactose, sucrose, cellobiose, and gentiobiose (Fig. 2.7). Disac-

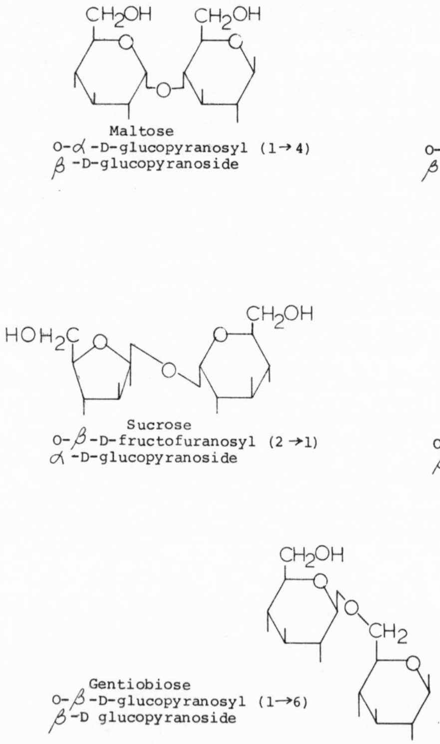

FIG. 2.7. Some important disaccharides.

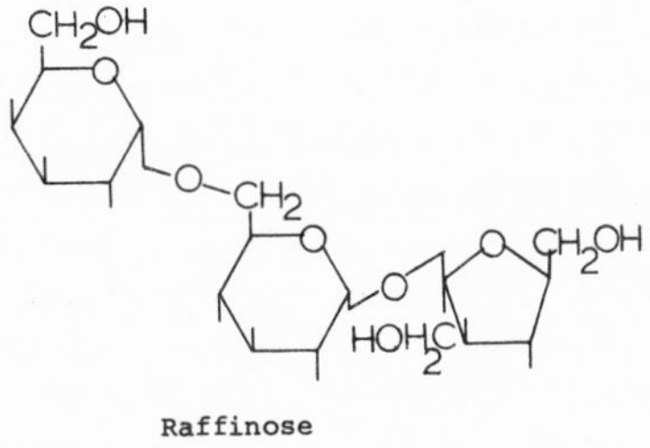

FIG. 2.8.   The structure of raffinose, O-α-D-galactopyranosyl (1 → 6) O-α-D-glucopyranosyl (1 → 2)β-D-fructofuranoside.

Raffinose

charides that have a free anomeric carbon are reducing sugars. Since sucrose has no free anomeric carbons, it does not have multiple conformational forms, and it is not a reducing sugar. Hydrolysis of sucrose, however, leads to multiple conformers and thus to optical rotation in a process called inversion. Sucrose is sometimes called invert sugar as a result. Lactose is the chief sugar in milk but is not found elsewhere in nature. Upon hydrolysis it yields free glucose and free galactose. Hydrolysis of maltose, cellobiose, or gentiobiose yields two glucose units. The differences in properties and metabolism of these disaccharides are due entirely to the differing linkages between the two glucosyl residues.

In assigning names to these compounds (and to any sugar larger than a monomer), the convention is to identify the compound starting from the left, indicating first what the position of the anomeric hydoxyl on the first unit is, then the name of this unit, then the carbons involved in the bond, then the configuration of the next anomeric carbon, and the name of this monomeric unit. This process continues until one runs out of units to name with the terminal unit being a furan- or pyranoside.

F. TRISACCHARIDES

There are many trisaccharides but two of the more well-studied ones are raffinose, which is abundant in sugar beets (Fig. 2.8), and melezitose found in the sap of pine trees. Melezitose is O-α-D-glucopyranosyl-(1→3)-O-β-D-fructofuranosyl-(2→1)-α-D-glucopyranoside.

G. SUMMARY

The monosaccharides may have a number of alterations at one or more of their hydroxyl positions. These alterations may result in amino sugars, sugar acids, deoxysugars, and sugar alcohols. Two very important monomer derivatives are muramic acid found in bacterial cell walls and N-acetylneuraminic acid found in cell coats of higher animals. Bacterial cell walls also depend on murein, teichoic acids, and other polysaccharide chains for their toughness. A number of disaccharides are important in nature; these include sucrose, cellobiose, lactose, maltose, and gentiobiose. Those disaccharides with at least one free anomeric carbon are reducing sugars. There are a number of trisaccharides as well, the most well known of which are raffinose from sugar beets and melezitose from pine sap.

REVIEW QUESTIONS

1. What are the systematic names for the following compounds?
   a. Lactose
   b. Maltose
   c. Sucrose
2. How would you determine whether a sample of sugar is maltose or sucrose using a chemical analysis?
3. What are the resultant products of C-1, C-1 and C-6, and C-6 oxidations?

BIBLIOGRAPHY

Dyson, R. 1978. Cell Biology, A Molecular Approach, 2nd Edition. Allyn and Bacon, Boston, Massachusetts.
Lehninger, A. 1975. Biochemistry, 2nd Edition. Worth Publishers, New York.
McGilvery, R., and Goldstein, G. 1979. Biochemistry, A Functional Approach, 2nd Edition. W. B. Saunders Co., Philadelphia, Pennsylvania.

3

Types of Complex Carbohydrates

A. INTRODUCTION AND DEFINITIONS

Upon complete hydrolysis polysaccharides yield monosaccharides or their derivatives. By convention a polysaccharide contains more than 10 monomeric units. Some polysaccharides are so large that they have molecular weights well into the millions. Glucose is the most common unit but polymers of mannose, fructose, galactose, xylose, and arabinose are frequent. Derivatives that are often found are glucosamine, galactosamine, glucuronic acid, N-acetylneuraminic acid, and N-acetylmuramic acid.

Polysaccharides are *homopolysaccharides* if they contain only one type of monomer and *heteropolysaccharides* if they contain a mixture of types. For example, glycogen, starch, amylopectin, and cellulose all are homopolysaccharides. A compound such as hyaluronic acid, on the other hand, is a heteropolysaccharide. Homopolysaccharides are named according to their repeating unit. They may be glucans, fructans, mannans, etc.

B. STORAGE POLYSACCHARIDES

The main storage forms of polysaccharides are glycogen in animal cells and starch in plant cells. Both are deposited as granules in cells. Starch can be found in one of two forms: α-amylose or amylopectin. Amylose consists of long unbranched chains of glucose attached to each other in α(1→4) linkages. These chains may be from 3000 to 500,000 molecular weight. α-Amylose readily forms hydrated micelles, and the chains form helical coils.

Amylopectin, on the other hand (which more closely resembles animal glycogen), is highly branched with 24–30 residues/branch. The chains have α(1→4) linkages but the branch points consist of α(1→6) linkages (Fig. 3.1). Amylopectin forms colloidal or micellar suspensions, and its molecular weight can be as high as 100 million. Amylose can be distinguished from amylopectin by the iodine test: amylose

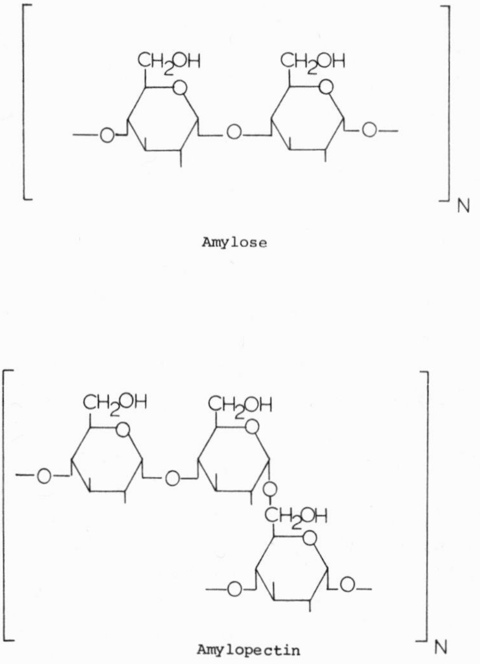

Amylose

Amylopectin

FIG. 3.1. Structures of amylose and amylopectin.

gives a deep blue color with iodine whereas amylopectin yields a red-violet color. The color obtained is believed to be due to a complex between the iodine and the helical coil of the polysaccharide and is dependent on the number of monomers in an unbranched section.

Glycogen is found to some extent in all animal cells but it is found in the largest quantities in skeletal muscle (1–2% of the muscle wet) and in liver (up to 10% of the liver wet weight under some conditions). On a fat-free basis, adipose tissue also has a relatively high glycogen content (about 1%). Glycogen is structurally similar to amylopectin but is more highly branched with only 8–12 residues in a linear sequence between branches. Therefore, it is a more compact molecule than amylopectin. It is found in cells in granules composed of subgranules. Also associated with these granules are enzymes of glycogen synthesis and degradation. Glycogen can be distinguished from amylose and amylopectin in that it gives a reddish brown color with iodine.

There are other storage polysaccharides. These include the *dextrans,* which are polymers of D-glucose with glycosidic linkages other than $\alpha(1{\rightarrow}4)$. The dextrans have important commercial use as chromatography supports and blood extenders. *Fructans* (levans) such as inulin, a $\beta(2{\rightarrow}1)$ polymer of fructose, are found in high concentration in Jerusalem artichokes and are especially useful in studies of renal function and blood volume. They give no color with iodine. Mannans are found in bacteria, yeasts, molds, and plants. Some of these complexes are so compact and so insoluble that they have been used to make very good buttons. Xylans and arabinans are abundant in plants. Galactomannans are elaborated by dermatophytes causing athlete's foot.

C. STRUCTURAL POLYSACCHARIDES

The most abundant animal polysaccharide is chitin. It is the major component of the exoskeletons of insects and crustacea. It is an N-acetyl-D-glucosamine $\beta(1 \rightarrow 4)$ homopolymer (Fig. 3.2). Increasing interest in chitin as a specialty material has arisen as the result of some of its properties (Austin *et al.* 1981). Chitin promotes wound healing and could be used as suture material if the problems involved in making filaments of it could be overcome. Microcrystalline chitin has also been added to animal feed, and used as binders and as thickening agents in cosmetics.

Cellulose is the most abundant polysaccharide on earth. Cotton is nearly pure cellulose. It is an ideal substance in conjunction with lignin to provide the rigid cell walls necessary to withstand the large osmotic pressure differences between the extracellular and intracellular compartments of plant cells. It is a linear polymer of glucoses linked $\beta(1 \rightarrow 4)$ and there are no branch points.

Partial hydrolysis of cellulose yields the disaccharide cellobiose. The molecular weight of cellulose ranges from 50,000 to as high as five million. Although cellulose is insoluble in water, it does have a high affinity for water. In plants, cellulose chains are arranged in bundles. Each bundle, having about 40 cellulose molecules, makes up the elementary fibril.

In a plant cell, the fibers form regular parallel arrays in crisscross layers "glued" together by three other polymeric materials. The first of these is hemicellulose, a term that describes a rather broad class of compounds. For the most part, hemicellulose is a polymer of pentoses, for example, D-xylose linked $\beta(1 \rightarrow 4)$ with D-arabinose and other sugars. The second polymeric material is pectin, a polymer of methyl-D-galacturonate, and the third is extensin, a glycoprotein similar to collagen with side chains of arabinose and galactose.

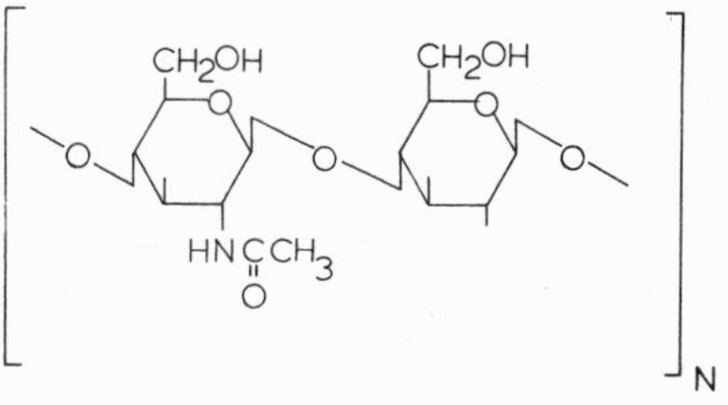

FIG. 3.2.   Chitin.

Among other structural polysaccharides are agar, alginic acid, gum arabic, and muropeptide (murein). Agar is composed of D- and L-galactoses which may be esterified with sulfate. D-Mannuronic acid is the primary component of alginic acid whereas gum arabic is made up of D-galactose and D-glucuronic acid residues. Muropeptide, which is found in bacterial cell walls, is a disaccharide of N-acetyl-D-glucosamine linked β(1→4) with N-acetylmuramic acid. The parallel side chains are cross-linked via peptide side chains linked covalently through alanine. The amino acid side chains are often composed of D-amino acids and thus are resistant to attack by mammalian peptide hydrolyzing enzymes. Lysozyme in tears, however, can attack the β(1→4) glycosidic linkages causing the bacterial cells (gram-positive) to swell and break.

The bacterial cell wall also contains teichoic acids (polymers of glycerol and ribitol linked by phosphodiester bridges) as well as other polysaccharides. The cell walls of gram-negative bacteria are somewhat more complex. One component found there is a lipopolysaccharide containing a repeating trisaccharide composed of two heptoses and one octulose.

D. MUCOPOLYSACCHARIDES

Mucopolysaccharides are incorporated in the "cell wall" equivalent of animals. They are *heteropolysaccharides* with usually two types of alternating monomers, one of which has an acidic group on it. In complexes with proteins they are called *mucins* or *mucoproteins*. These are sticky, slippery, and jellylike compounds that function as intercellular lubricants and as flexible cement in the body.

The most abundant of the mucopolysaccharides is *hyaluronic acid*, which is found in cell coats and in the extracellular ground substance of the connective tissue of vertebrates. It is also found in the synovial fluid of joints and the vitreous humor of the eye. It a linear polymer composed of D-glucuronic acid linked β(1→3) with N-acetyl-D-glucosamine, which is then linked β(1→4) with the next D-glucuronate (Fig. 3.3).

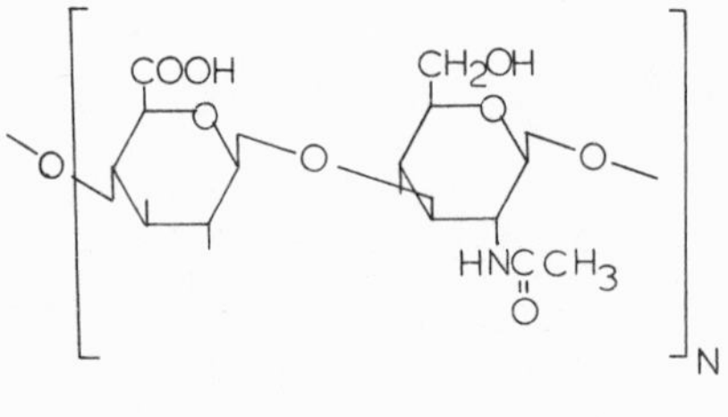

FIG. 3.3.   Hyaluronic acid.

Chondroitin is similar to hyaluronic acid except that it contains
N-acetyl-D-galactosamine instead of N-acetyl-D-glucosamine. There is
little free chondroitin in the body, but the sulfated forms are widely
distributed in cell coats, bone, cornea, skin, and connective tissue of
vertebrates. There are several types of chondroitin sulfate. Condroitin
sulfates A and C both contain D-glucuronic acid and 2-amino-2-de-
oxy-D-galactose, acetyl, and sulfate residues in equimolar quantities.
Type A has the sulfate in the 4 position and type C has it in the 6
position. Chondroitin sulfate B contains iduronic rather than glucuronic acid.

The structure of *heparin* is not so clearly defined. It does, however,
have equimolar amounts of D-glucuronic acid and 2-amino-2-deoxy-
glucose. In this case the amino sugars are N- sulfated rather than N-
acetylated. Heparin is an endogenous anticoagulant and antilipaemic
agent. It is mostly found bound to tissue protein and is highest in
concentration in the liver capsule, in mast cells, and in cells lining the
circulatory system. In mast cells heparin is found associated with
granules that also contain histamine, proteases, and Zn^{2+}.

E. GLYCOPROTEINS

Proteins that contain carbohydrate covalently linked to protein are
called *glycoproteins*. If the carbohydrate content is high relative to the
protein content then they are often referred to as *proteoglycans*. There
are three classes of linkages between the carbohydrate and an amino
acid of the protein portion (Fig. 3.4). One type has an N-glucosyl link to
the amide nitrogen of asparagine. A second type has a glycosidic bond
between N-acetylgalactosamine and a serine or threonine hydroxyl,
and a third has an attachment of the carbohydrate to the protein via
the hydroxyl of hydroxylysine (e.g., collagen). The glycosidic linkage to
serine or threonine predominates in mucous secretion glycoproteins.
The glycosidic linkage to hydroxylysine occurs predominately in the
fibrillar collagens. Other linkages have been found such as between

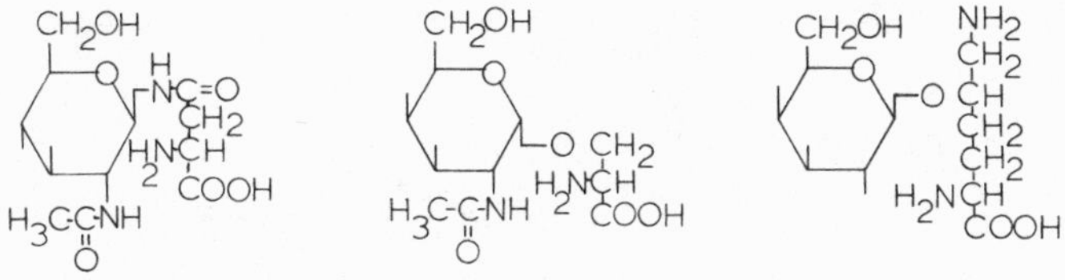

1	2	3
N-glycosyl link to asparagine	Glycosidic link to serine or threonine	Glycosidic link to hydroxylysine

FIG. 3.4.   Major glycopeptide linkages.

L-fucose and L-threonine, a thioglycosidic linkage between D-glucose and L-cysteine, and links between arabinose or galactose and hydroxyproline in plant cells. Certainly, there may be additional linkages as well.

Glycoproteins play an enormous number of important roles in the body. There are a number of blood glycoproteins such as the immunoglobulins and fibrinogen. Hormones, such as follicle stimulating hormone and thyroid stimulating hormone, are also in this class as well as many enzymes, including ribonuclease A and pepsin. Other proteins, for example, avidin, ovalbumin, and collagen, are also members of the glycoprotein family. This list is only representative; in reality there are a great many members of this group. One of the very important roles of glycoproteins is in cellular contact and recognition phenomenon. This area has been receiving increasing attention of late because of the implications for the field of tumor growth and immunology.

F. GLYCOLIPIDS

The glycolipids usually receive more attention in discussions of lipids than in discussions about carbohydrates. Many of the glycolipids are found in nerve tissue. There are several classes of glycolipids (Fig. 3.5). *Glycosyldiacylglycerols* are composed of a diacylglycerol in which the unesterified third hydroxyl of the glycerol is hooked to a monosaccharide (or a di- or trisaccharide) in a glycosidic linkage. The *neutral glycosphingolipids* may contain one sugar (*cerebroside*), a disaccharide

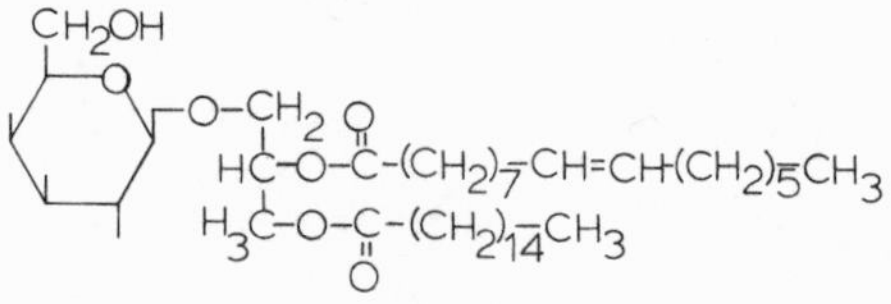

FIG. 3.5.   Glycolipid classes.

1. Glycosyldiacyl glycerol

2. Neutral glycospingolipids

Galactose β-ceramide	Cerebroside
Disaccharide-ceramide	Dihexoside
Trisaccharide-ceramide	Trihexoside
Tetrasaccharide-ceramide	Tetrahexoside

3. Acidic glycosphingolipids (gangliosides)
   Sailic acid (2→3) Gal β (1→4) Glu 1-β-
   ceramide (GM^3)

(*dihexoside*) or a trisaccharide (*trihexoside*) in a β linkage with ce-ramide, which is sphingosine conjugated by an amide linkage to a monounsaturated fatty acid. These compounds are named on the basis of the sugar that is attached to the ceramide, e.g., if galactose is hooked to ceramide then it would be called a galactocerebroside. Sometimes these compounds have sulfate esters at the 3 position of galactose and are then known as *sulfatides* which are important to neural tissue and are also found on cell surfaces where their nonpolar lipid tails can intereact with the lipid bilayer of the cell membrane leaving the polar carbohydrate head to stick out above the cell surface.

The *gangliosides* all contain N-acetylneuraminic acid (*sialic acid*) in various amounts. Most gangliosides have a glucose residue attached directly to the ceramide but the rest of the carbohydrate chain can be made of branched and unbranched residues of galactose, N-acetyl-galactosamine, and sialic acid. More than 20 gangliosides are known and are identified by a large G then a subscript letter and number, e.g., G_{M3}, G_{M1}, G_{D1}, and G_{T1}.

The gangliosides play a number of important roles. They make up 6% of the total lipid of the brain's gray matter and are found in high concentration especially in nerve endings. They may also be involved in neurotransmitter receptor sites. In nonneural locations they are involved in tissue recognition, blood group specificity, and tissue im-munity, and may have special roles in cancer. Errors in the metabo-lism of these compounds are especially important in several usually fatal genetic diseases such as Tay–Sachs disease.

G. SUMMARY

The complex carbohydrates may be composed of the same or differ-ent repeating units and are known accordingly as homo- or hetero-polysaccharides. These compounds serve as fuel storage or structural elements in the cell. They may also have specialized functions as inter-cellular lubricants, anticoagulants, or cell–cell recognition factors.

The energy storage polysaccharides (glycogen and starch) and two of the major structural carbohydrates (cellulose and chitin) are homo-polysaccharides. Three major classes of heteropolysaccharides are mucopolysaccharides, glycoproteins, and glycolipids. In the latter two classes, carbohydrates are attached to either amino acids or lipids, respectively.

REVIEW QUESTIONS

1. Define
   a. Homopolysaccharide
   b. Heteropolysaccharide
   c. Mucopolysaccharide

2. How do amylose, glycogen, and amylopectin differ from each other? How do they react in the presence of iodine?
3. How do neutral glycospingolipids differ from gangliosides?

BIBLIOGRAPHY

Albers, G. Siegel, R. Katzman, and B. Agranoff (Editors). 1972. Basic Neurochemistry. Little, Brown and Company, Boston, Massachusetts.

Austin, P., Brine, C., Castle, J., and Zikakis, J. 1981. Chitin: new facets of research. Science 212, 749.

Brady, R. 1973. Hereditary fat-metabolism diseases. Sci. Am. *229,* 88–97.

Horowitz, M., and Pigman, W. (Editors). 1982. The Glycoconjugates, Vol. 3, Glycoproteins, Glycolipids and Proteoglycans. Academic Press New York.

McGilvery, R., and Goldstein, G. 1979. Biochemistry, A Functional Approach. W. B. Saunders, Philadelphia, Pennsylvania.

Sharon, N. 1974. Glycoproteins. Sci. Am. *230,* 541–574.

Sharon, N., and Hill, R. 1982. Glycoproteins. *In* The Proteins, 3rd Edition, Vol. 5, pp. 1–144. H. Neurath and R. Hill (Editors). Academic Press, New York.

Staneloni, R., and Leloir, L. 1982. The biosynthetic pathway of asparagine linked oligosaccharides of glycoproteins. CRC Crit. Rev. Biochem. *12,* 289–326.

Wagh, P., and Bahl, O. 1981. Sugar residues on proteins. CRC Crit. Rev. Biochem. *10,* 307–377.

Part II

Digestion and Absorption of Carbohydrates

4

Digestion of Simple Carbohydrates

A. PERCEPTION OF SWEET TASTE

Carbohydrate makes up as much as 80% of the human diet in some countries: in the United States about half of the calories are supplied by carbohydrate. The proportion of simple sugars has been increasing in Western diets. The desire for sweet taste seems to be universal and appears at birth rather than being acquired. Not only do we consume sugar intentionally for caloric expenditure but sweeteners are added to such products as mouthwash and medicines to improve their acceptability.

The ability to taste various substances is associated with specialized organs called taste buds. In lower animals, such as fish, taste buds are found not only in the mouth but in some species they are dispersed over the entire body as well. In the adult human, taste buds are confined to the tongue and palate, but in the fetus they are found on the lips, pharynx, and epiglottis as well. These organs appear about the same time that the fetus starts swallowing, that is, at 3–4 months of gestational age. The ability to taste "sweet" is greatest at the tip of the tongue.

Why do some compounds taste sweet and others do not? Several theories have been reviewed by Birch and Lee (1979). A number of theories have been offered over the years including that sweetness is a function of the number of hydroxyl groups on a compound. Many subsequent studies have demonstrated that this is not true (Birch and Lee 1979). No unifying hypothesis was available, however, until 1963 when Shallenberger proposed that the spatial orientation of certain electronegative atoms triggered a sweet sensation. It was thought that for a compound to taste sweet, it must have an electronegative atom with a covalently attached hydrogen and another covalent atom within a 3 Å distance (Shallenberger and Acree 1967). This alone, however, is necessary but insufficient to predict the sweetness of a compound. A subsequent modification of the hypothesis was that a third interacting substituent was necessary.

The cells involved in taste sensations are highly innervated. Although the nerve fibers themselves can respond to a variety of taste sensations, the ability to discriminate sweet tastes, for example, is due to the presence of lectins, which are associated with the outer surface of the taste buds. *Lectins* are carbohydrate binding proteins. Lectins are glycoproteins and are capable of recognizing with great specificity a variety of different carbohydrates. Although lectins serve a variety of other functions associated with carbohydate binding in both plants and animals, binding of carbohydrate to them is necessary for the transmission of a nerve impulse to the brain which indicates that a sugar is being ingested.

In mammals, sucrose causes a greater neural discharge than any other natural sweetener. There are sites (lectins) that are specific for different sugars. For example, glucose and fructose can be differentiated. To gerbils and humans α-D-glucopyranose is sweeter than β-D-glucopyranose. On the cow tongue, there are separate sites for glucose, fructose, and sucrose (Jakinovich 1979).

The degree to which compounds are sweet depends to some extent on the local environment. Compounds in the dry state are not as sweet as in dilute solution. Presumably, a solution allows greater access of the sugar to the lectin. Sweetness also depends on pH and the presence of other compounds.

The sensation of a sweet taste is probably part of the body's "prepriming" mechanism for the initiation of the processes for digestion, absorption, and utilization of dietary carbohydrate. Prepriming aids in maintaining whole body carbohydrate homeostasis. Other events that also undoubtedly contribute to homeostasis are the thought, sight, and smell of some particular food. For some the mental vision of a richly frosted chocolate layer cake or a piece of creamy divinity is sufficient to excite the gustatory response, stimulating salivary secretions and creating hunger pangs as well.

B. ROLE OF SALIVARY GLANDS

Although no digestion of simple carbohydrates occurs in the mouth or esophagus, a process does occur here that is important to digestion. The salivary glands secrete fluid to (1) lubricate food for chewing and swallowing, (2) provide solvation for food for better interaction with taste receptors, and (3) dilute noxious tastes. In man 1–2 liters/day of salivary secretion are produced, and the volume is much higher than this in ruminants (4 liters/day for sheep and up to 100 liters/day for cows). In ruminants, salivary secretion serves also to buffer the rumen contents and maintain rumen fluid volume.

Different salivary glands produce different secretions. The parotid gland produces a secretion devoid of mucin. The submaxillary and sublingual glands secrete material high in mucins containing neuraminic acid and fucose.

The Na^+/K^+ ratio in salivary secretion is about 18/1. If an animal is fistulated to prevent the ingestion of this secretion, 400–600 meq of Na^+ is depleted. This leads to a collapse of the extracellular fluid volume and ultimately to death. During Ramadan, the ninth month of the Mohammedan year, fasting between sunrise and sunset is observed. Neither food nor water is permitted. The most devout spit rather than swallow their own saliva. In some cases this leads to such severe fluid and sodium depletion that death ensues. The Na^+/K^+ ratio of saliva is regulated by the mineralocorticoids of the adrenal cortex. Salivary secretion is virtually abolished during sleep, dehydration, anxiety, or severe mental effort. A walk across the desert or a final exam can produce the same result. Salivation is increased by chewing and is proportional to the size of the bolus and to the amount of taste sensation. Understandably, a strongly flavored food like lemon drops produces a large amount of saliva. Metabolically, resting salivary glands are sixfold more active than resting skeletal muscle.

C. ABSORPTION OF SIMPLE CARBOHYDRATES

In the nonruminant animal, most of the absorption of simple sugars occurs in the upper small intestine. The rate at which simple sugars are released from the stomach is controlled by a negative feedback mechanism involving receptors in the upper intestine and by motility of the stomach. The intestine is osmoresponsive to sugar so a load of monosaccharide into the gut will cause the water balance to shift. When too much sugar gets out of the stomach at once then dumping syndrome may occur: water is drawn to the gut and osmotic diarrhea is the result. In general, the stomach empties at a rate that supplies a constant amount of calories to the intestines. Hence a high fat diet slows stomach emptying. There is apparently some discrimination by the emptying mechanism, however, which is controlled by the type of monosaccharide in the stomach. Figure 4.1 illustrates that glucose

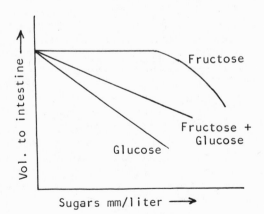

FIG. 4.1. Effect of various monosaccharides on stomach emptying.

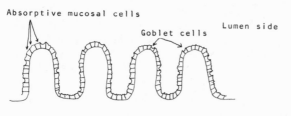

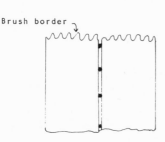

FIG. 4.2. (Top) The intestinal wall. (Bottom) Enlarged mucosal cells showing the junction between the cells.

retards stomach emptying to a greater extent than does fructose. It has been estimated that the absorptive capacity per day for the human intestine, all other considerations aside, amounts to 5374 g/day for glucose and 4837 g/day for fructose. Unless one is exceedingly gluttinous, however, this ultimate capability is never tapped.

How can the intestine manage this remarkable feat? The area of absorption in the small intestine is composed of absorptive mucosal cells and mucus-secreting goblet cells that line projections called villi (Fig. 4.2). The oldest cells are at the tips of the villi. These cells have the greatest absorptive efficiency. The absorptive cells have a hairy projection-like surface on the lumen side called the microvilli or brush border. This results in an enormous total surface area. In large mammals there are also 8–10 mm folds in the intestine which further increases the absorptive area. The brush border has 2×10^5 projections per square millimeter. The membrane of the microvilli has a thicker than usual carbohydrate coat called the *glycocalyx*. The mucosal cells live only 3–4 days before being sloughed off. The villi are very well supplied with blood and lymphatic vessels and are innervated. There is a junctional barrier between the cells which allows water to pass but not large molecules so it is not a tight junction. On the lumen side there is a layer of quiescent material close to the brush border. It is composed of gut contents (nutrients, etc.). This layer, the *unstirred layer,* is out of the stream of mixing and propulsion that goes on more toward the center of the lumen. Literature on the structure and physiology of the intestine has been recently reviewed by Moog (1981).

Glucose and galactose are absorbed across the gut wall by *active transport* whereas fructose goes across by *facilitated diffusion*. Active transport means that the process *is energy requiring, involves a specific carrier* and *can occur against a concentration gradient*. If one were to poison gut cells with a blocker of oxidative phosphorylation, then transport of glucose and galactose would also cease. Other criteria for active transport are that the transport system be *saturatable* (rate of transport does not increase infinitely with an increase in glucose concentration) and that there is *competitive inhibition* of the transport system by analogs of the substrate. Active transport of sugar is necessary when there is a higher serosal concentration of a sugar than there is in the lumen. This might be particularly true for glucose where the blood levels are 4–5 mM and levels in some diets might not be that high.

Facilitated diffusion, on the other hand, is *not* an energy requiring process and so it can only proceed down a concentration gradient. There is an actual carrier involved, however, so the system is saturatable and will show competitive inhibition. Since fructose is very effectively trapped from the bloodstream by the liver, there is virtually no circulating fructose in the bloodstream. Therefore, no active transport system is required for fructose since absorption would nearly always be down a concentration gradient.

Some details of the specificity and nature of the active transport system for glucose and galactose have been determined. Similar sugars with modifications around the C-1 carbon can be transported unless the substituents are too large. Gold thioglucose (—S—Au), for example, cannot be transported by the active transport system. Modifications to the C-2 position impair transport especially if the hydroxyl is involved. Changes in the C-2 hydrogen have less severe consequences as long as the group is not too large. Substitution with large groups at any other position also impairs transport. C-3 and C-4 epimers of glucose (allose, and galactose, respectively) are readily transported, but sugars with a C-3 and C-4 combined rearrangement (gulose) are not transported at all. Xylose is the chief pentose that is actively absorbed.

The exact nature of the glucose carrier is unclear. However, it is known to be a protein complex connected to the Na^+/K^+ pump. Na^+ is required for glucose uptake, but the reverse is not true. Glucose or galactose cannot attach to the carrier until it is preloaded with Na^+. Some cases of glucose malabsorption have been shown to be due to a reduced number of carriers. Some glucose will cross the mucosal cell barrier by simple diffusion if the gut glucose concentration is sufficiently high. Sorbitol, xylitol, and mannose are absorbed strictly by passive diffusion.

Active transport is actually not one process but a combination of three. There is an unstirred layer of material immediately contiguous to the mucosal cells on the lumen side through which glucose must first diffuse. Then the actual transport occurs. Finally, there is extrusion of glucose from the cell to the serosal side into the interstitial fluid. The diffusion part of this process is regulated by the law of diffusion:

$$J = D/d \, (C_1 - C_2)$$

where J is the diffusion rate which is proportional to the diffusion constant of the sugar (D) divided by the thickness of the unstirred layer (d) times the difference in the concentration of the sugar in the bulk phase (C_1) and its concentration at the interface between the cell and the unstirred layer (C_2).

In the nonruminant, most of the absorbable simple sugars cross the mucosal cell barrier intact. Only about 10% of the glucose crossing is used by the mucosal cell itself. In the ruminant, this is not the case. There is a large microbial and protozoal population in the rumen fluid. The contents of the rumen are maintained anaerobically at 39°C and pH 5–7. Maintenance of pH is aided by large volumes (80–100 liters/day for cows) of alkaline saliva. Any simple sugars in the diet are rapidly fermented by rumen organisms to lactate, volatile fatty acids, CO_2, or methane or are used by these microbes to make their own cellular components. Therefore, virtually no dietary simple sugar would be left for absorption by the animal. Ruminants do, however, have a similar capacity to nonruminants in their upper intestinal tracts for absorption of monosaccharides, and mechanistically the processes are the same. In ruminants, however, this capacity is very rarely utilized because of the extensive fermentation of monosaccharides that occurs in the rumen.

D. SUMMARY

Digestion and absorption of simple carbohydrates occur in the small intestine in nonruminants. Although ruminants have the same intestinal absorptive mechanisms as nonruminants, these mechanisms are rarely used because microbial fermentation in the rumen converts the simple sugars to lactate, proprionate, acetate, CO_2, methane, and other products. Prepriming the body for carbohydrate metabolism is the result of the ability to perceive a sweet taste due to lectins in the taste buds. Although monosaccharides are neither digested nor absorbed in the stomach, there is regulation of gastric emptying by various sugars. Once the sugar reaches the upper gastrointestinal tract it is absorbed either by active transport, facilitated diffusion, or simple diffusion. Only about 10% of the sugar transported to the mucosal cell is used by the cell; the rest crosses to the bloodstream.

REVIEW QUESTIONS

1. Define:
   a. Lectin
   b. Brush border
   c. Active transport.
2. What are the functions of saliva?
3. What is the fate of dietary glucose in nonruminants? In ruminants?

BIBLIOGRAPHY

Birch, G., and Lee, C. 1979. The theory of sweetness. *In* Developments in Sweeteners, Vol. 1. C. Hough, K. Parker, and A. Vlitos (Editors). Applied Science Publ., London.

Church, D. (Editor) 1979. Digestive Physiology and Nutrition of Ruminants, Vol. 2. O and B Books, Corvallis, Oregon.

Davenport, H. 1977. Physiology of the Digestive Tract. Yearbook Medical Publishers, Chicago, Illinois.

Jakinovich, W. 1979. The specificity of sugar taste responses in the gerbil. *In* Carbohydrate Protein Interactions. ACS Symp. Vol. 88. Am. Chem. Soc. Washington D.C.

Koldovsky, O. 1972. Hormonal and dietary factors in the development of digestion and absorption. *In* Nutrition and Development. M. Winick (Editor). J. Wiley & Sons, New York.

McDonald, P., Edwards, R., and Greenhalgh, J. 1973. Animal Nutrition. Longmans, London.

Moog, F. 1981. The lining of the small intestine. Sci. Am. *245*, 154–176.

Shallenberger, R. 1976. Taste and bioavailability of sugars as related to structure. *In* Carbohydrate Metabolism. C. Berdanier (Editor). J. Wiley & Sons, New York.

Shallenberger, R., and Acree, T. 1967. Molecular theory of sweet taste. Nature *216*, 480–483.

5

Digestion of More Complex Carbohydrates

A. DISACCHARIDES

Virtually no digestion of disaccharides or oligosaccharides occurs in the mouth, esophagus, or stomach. In nonruminants it all occurs in the upper small intestine. The hydrolytic activity, however, is not found in the lumen of the gut but instead is found associated with the mucosal cells in the brush borders and terminal web. The highest activities are found in the midjejunal and upper ileal regions. Any oligosaccharidase activity that is found within the gut lumen itself is merely from desquamated cells.

There are a number of enzymes that catalyze the breakdown of disaccharides and oligosaccharides. The breakdown is necessary because under normal circumstances disaccharides cannot be absorbed. Any appearance of intact dietary disaccharides in circulating blood is due to absorption where there are microlesions in the mucosal cell wall since the normal junctions between the mucosal cells are not able to allow such a large molecule to pass.

Among the types of enzyme activities located in mucosal cells are maltase, lactase, isomaltase, and sucrase. *Maltase* hydrolyzes maltose and maltotriose to glucose, which is then absorbed via active transport on the glucose carrier. *Lactase* catalyzes the cleavage of lactose to equimolar amounts of galactose and glucose. Both of these monosaccharides then cross the gut wall on the glucose carrier. *Sucrase,* sometimes called *invertase* hydrolyzes sucrose to yield one glucose and one fructose. Fructose then crosses the mucosal cell barrier by facilitated diffusion. Sucrase can also act on maltose. *Isomaltase,* also called oligo-1,6-glucosidase or α-dextrinase, breaks down branched dextrins to glucose and maltose. The maltose is then further degraded by maltase. Other hydrolytic activities toward carbohydrates are also found in the brush borders. These include enzymes that attack cellobiose, α-glycerophosphate, hexosediphosphates, ATP, and other polyphosphates.

In most species hydrolysis of disaccharides is faster than absorption of the products. Thus, absorption is the rate-limiting step in the digestion process. The exception to this is lactose digestion where the activity of lactase may be lower than the ability of the gut to absorb the products. Maltose and sucrose are hydrolyzed at approximately the same rate, but lactose digestion is only half as fast as these two. There has been some controversy about the speed of absorption of glucose compared to fructose. In man, glucose appears to be absorbed 3–6 times faster than fructose. The rate of fructose absorption, however, is dependent on the concentration of fructose in the lumen since its absorption into the body is by facilitated diffusion. Thus, there is no advantage to feeding monosaccharides over disaccharides or vice versa because portal concentrations of monosaccharides will be the same in either case and the rate-limitation is on absorption and not on hydrolysis. The sites of absorption seem to be independent of meal composition. Regardless of the form of the food an animal ingests, the absorption of the ultimate end products always occurs on the same carriers in the upper small intestine.

In the fetus, age is the determinant for appearance of oligosaccharidases in the gut. Lactase, maltase, and sucrase activity can be found in the gut relatively early in gestation. Lactase, activity, however, does not peak until close to term. This is consistent with the metabolic needs of the mammal, since before birth, the fetus relies on blood glucose from the mother and during the postnatal period the neonate uses lactose from milk. Some animals, such as sea lion pups, have no oligosaccharidases and get osmotic diarrhea when fed lactose or sucrose. This is not a problem, however, since sea lion milk does not contain lactose or any other disaccharide.

B. POLYSACCHARIDES

Although digestion of disaccharides occurs as the result of brush border enzymes, digestion of starch occurs in a different way. The initial phase of digestion begins in the mouth as a result of salivary amylase, which is the major enzyme secreted by the salivary glands. Not all animals secrete salivary amylase as shown in Table 5.1. It is

TABLE 5.1. Salivary Amylase Secretion in Various Species

Secreted by	Not secreted by
Man (primates)	Horses
Pigs	Cats
Rats	Dogs
Squirrels	Fowls
Ruminants[a]	

[a] Although ruminants have detectable oral amylase activity, its origin is nasolabial.

not surprising, perhaps, that cats do not possess this enzyme since cats are predominately carnivores, and their diets would not ordinarily contain much starch.

The amylase found in saliva is an endoamylase which splits $\alpha(1\rightarrow4)$ glycosidic linkages *within* the chain. It is not a terminal amylase. The pH optimum for this enzyme is 6.9. Chloride ions, normally supplied in the saliva, are also necessary for optimum activity of this enzyme. The products of this reaction are maltose, maltotriose, and a mixture of dextrins containing $\alpha(1\rightarrow4)$ and $\alpha(1\rightarrow6)$ linkages. The duration of action, and hence the degree to which salivary amylase contributes to starch digestion, depends to a large extent on how long the pH stays high. If the food stays for a long time in the mouth or esophagus or if the pH of the stomach does not drop rapidly, then salivary amylase can contribute substantially to starch digestion. For those who gulp food and suffer immediate heartburn, it is unlikely that salivary amylase is very effective. The only digestion of starch that occurs in the stomach is the result of salivary amylase activity present before the pH drops so low that the enyme is no longer active. In many species, salivary amylase does not play a quantitatively important role in starch digestion.

Raw starch is not very digestible. Cooked starch, on the other hand, is fully digestible. Depending upon the source of starch, the concentration of amylose [all $\alpha(1\rightarrow4)$ linkages] and amylopectin [$\alpha(1\rightarrow4)$ and $\alpha(1\rightarrow6)$ linkages] will vary. Typical U.S. cornstarch is about 74% amylopectin and 24% amylose as commercially isolated. Starch granules are not readily hydrolyzed enzymatically until they are first partially broken down by heat. When suspensions of starch granules are heated, the granules swell taking up water and causing the polymers to become more accessible to enzymes.

The gut amylases are responsible for most of the digestion of starch in nonruminants. The first of these is α-amylase which attacks interior $\alpha(1\rightarrow4)$ linkages yielding the α-anomeric form of the sugar. The products are maltose, maltotriose, and α-limit dextrins (short chains that cannot be further degraded) containing an $\alpha(1\rightarrow6)$ linkage. The smallest limit dextrin is at least four monomers.

The amylase in the upper small intestine is pancreatic in origin arriving at the gut via the pancreatic duct. Amylase, like other proteins designed for export, is packaged in granules in the secretory cells of the pancreas. Upon stimulation, these granules are discharged from the cell, releasing amylase into the collecting ducts. Cholecystokinin–pancreozymin (CCK-PZ) and vagus nerve stimulation both cause increased release of amylase. Secretin also aids in this process by stimulating the flow of pancreatic juice and particularly the concentration of bicarbonate, which is necessary to maintain the 6.9 optimum pH for pancreatic amylase activity. Pancreatic amylase is similar to salivary amylase in that it also requires chloride ion for activity. The appearance of gut amylase corresponds roughly with the inclusion of starch in the diet. Hence, neonatal mammals existing only on milk will have relatively low amylase activity. Only around the time of weaning will amylase activity rise.

Ruminants are quite efficient at hydrolyzing starch in the rumen. Rumen amylase is mostly of bacterial origin and comes from *Bacteriodes amylophilus, Streptococcus bovis,* and *Succinimonas amylolytica.* The pancreatic amylase content in ruminants is relatively low. This is not surprising since little starch would ever arrive intact at the upper part of the tract in a ruminant.

There are some exoamylases as well. One of these is β-amylase which cleaves off monomers starting at the terminal nonreducing end. It cannot cleave α(1→6) linkages. This enzyme is found only in plants and microorganisms. Its presence in microorganisms in the lower gastrointestinal tract could contribute to some starch digestion in the lower gut for any starch excaping the upper tract. In ruminants it could be quite important if it is present in rumen microorganisms. The ultimate product of starch digestion in nonruminants is glucose via maltose and isomaltose which is absorbed as previously described. In ruminants, the glucose serves as a nutrient source for the rumen microorganism ending up primarily as volatile fatty acids and lactic acid.

C. CELLULOSE

Nonruminant mammals have no capacity to digest cellulose in the small intestine although the microflora in the large intestine may be able to digest significant quantities of cellulose depending on the duration of time the fecal matter stays in the colon and the types of microorganisms in the gut. The large intestine is in many ways similar to the rumen. Fermentation products can be absorbed into the animal from this site.

Ruminant mammals, on the other hand, are quite good at digesting cellulose. The digestive tract of a ruminant is substantially different than that of a nonruminant. It is composed, from front to back, of the mouth, esophagus, reticulum, rumen, omasum, abomasum, duodenum, small intestine, cecum, colon, and rectum. The reticulum and rumen although separate entities can be considered as one structural unit and together comprise 80–85% of the total stomach capacity. The abomasum is the true glandular stomach. The rumen has a high moisture content, a large bacterial and protozoal population, and a strong musculature for agitation of the contents. The types of bacteria and protozoa found in the rumen are dependent on the composition of the diet. The temperature is about 39°C (cow) and the pH is maintained from 5–7 with the aid of large quantities of alkaline saliva. No hydrolytic enzymes are secreted by the *animal* into this compartment. Bacterial concentrations of 10^{10}–10^{11} per gram and protozoa of 10^5–10^6 per gram are normal. A 500 kg cow has nearly 70 liters of rumen content (about 15% of the total body weight).

The movement of material through the rumen is a controlled process. The rumen has two layers: a lower liquid phase composed of fine particles and an upper phase containing the coarser material. In animals fed high concentrate diets, there may not be distinguishable layers. The coarse material is regurgitated, chewed 40 times or so, then reswallowed. This is known as *ruminating* or cud chewing. The coarseness of the food determines the amount of time spent in rumination. Grazing cattle spend about one-half their waking time eating and one-half ruminating. Actually, rumination is not restricted to ruminants. Many of the great apes and large cats in zoos can be observed to perform the same action. Although the practice is not aesthetically pleasing, it may serve a useful purpose in that an animal can swallow his food quickly while it is available then move on to a place of greater safety to decide at leisure how much of what was consumed will be reeaten.

Contractions of the rumen also wash fine particles on through to the omasum where water is resorbed. Then the particles transit to the true stomach where gastric juices are secreted by the animal. Emptying of the true stomach is controlled in a way that is remarkably similar to that of nonruminants. Bicarbonate is a potent stimulator of emptying whereas fat delays emptying. Gastrin stimulates gastric acid secretion. Volatile fatty acids, the products of saccharide digestion by microorganisms in the rumen, also play a role in potentiating release of the hormones that control emptying and motility.

Among the complex carbohydrates digestible in the rumen, besides cellulose, are pectin and hemicellulose. Cellulose is digested by the enzyme cellulase which has a broad pH optimum of 4–7.5. The change in pH with various types of diets leads to a change in the pattern of carbohydrate fermentation, not because the optima of the lytic enzymes change but because the type of microflora change. Some of the cellulose fermenting bacteria are *Bacteriodes succinogenes, Butyrivibrio fibrosolvens,* and *Ruminococcus flavefaciens.* Some of the oligotrich protozoa are also capable of digesting cellulose.

Cellulose is seldom a free dietary component. In nature it is associated with lignin (lignocellulose) and hemicellulose. These three components make up the cell wall of plants. Lignin is an aromatic polymer (Fig. 5.1). Its concentration is low in young plants and high in mature

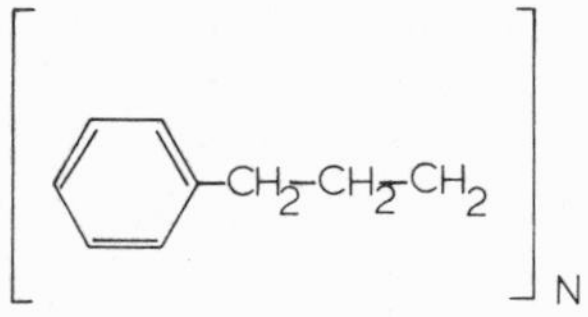

FIG. 5.1.   Lignin.

plants (15%), especially woody plants. Phenylpropane is the basic repeating unit. The ring may contain one or more —OCH_3 groups. Lignin is indigestible enzymatically and is also chemically resistant. It may act as a physical barrier to cellulose digestion (MacAllister 1979). Therefore, grinding cellulosic type materials to small size improves the digestibility because cellulase can come into closer contact with cellulose in the plant material although there is a lower limit to particle size for maximum digestion. If particle size gets too small, the particles do not stay in the rumen long enough for the cellulolytic bacteria to break down the cellulose. Cellulose can be from 25 to 90% digestible depending on its form. Although there seems to be a requirement for a small amount of readily digestible carbohydrate to stimulate lignocellulose digestion, too much depresses lignocellulose utilization.

D. HEMICELLULOSE

Hemicellulose makes up 10–30% of roughages commonly found in ruminant feed. The hemicellulose content of grass rises as the grass ages. Hemicellulose is really a heterogeneous class of modified and unmodified hexose and pentose polymers. Xylans are probably the most prevalent and widely distributed of the hemicelluloses. Mannans, galactans, and arabanans are also important. The bacteria *Bacteriodes ruminicola, Butyrivibrio fibrosolvens,* and *Lachnospira multiparus* are all efficient hemicellulolytic bacteria. Bacteria that metabolize cellulose can also metabolize hemicellulose but the reverse is not usually true. The enzymes that degrade this class of compound are xylanases, mannanases, etc. The hemicellulases are all endocellulases, that is, they attack the linkages interior to the chain.

The change in hemicellulose digestion that one observes with increasing age of the plant material could be due to the change in lignin content. As lignin concentration increases the physical barrier that it causes limits hemicellulose digestion. Another factor could be the change in hemicellulose composition. If the composition changed from a high proportion of xylans to a high arabinan content, the digestibility would drop drastically. As with cellulose, the products of hemicellulose metabolism are volatile fatty acids or lactate. Some hemicellulose digestion can occur in the colon, but this does not contribute a large percentage to the total hemicellulose.

Ruminants play a very important role in the food chain. For the most part (in the wild) they do not compete for the same foodstuffs as nonruminant animals. Ruminants can get useful energy from grasses and woody materials and ultimately turn it into high quality meat and milk for man and his pets. One has the added advantage of the byproducts as well: leather for shoes, bone meal, wool, etc. Since man can derive little benefit from grasses (besides that of the exercise involved in mowing one's lawn), the ruminant is a vital energy link between plants and nonruminant animals.

E. SUMMARY

In nonruminants, disaccharides are digested by intestinal mucosal cell hydrolases, and the resultant monosaccharides are absorbed into the mucosal cell by active transport or facilitated diffusion depending on the type of sugar. All of these hydrolases are associated with the mucosal cells themselves and are found in the lumen only as a product of sloughed off mucosal cells. Starch digestion starts with salivary amylase but in most species is accomplished predominately by pancreatic amylase secreted into the lumen of the gut. Ruminant animals ferment most sugars and starch to form volatile fatty acids, lactate, methane, and CO_2. By virtue of the rumen microbial population, ruminants also can readily metabolize cellulose and hemicellulose depending on the content of lignin in the plant material and several other factors. The nonruminant colon may also function somewhat like the rumen. There may be significant cellulose digestion and the products of fermentation can be absorbed.

REVIEW QUESTIONS

1. Where are the disaccharides found?
2. What are the end products of amylase digestion of starch in the ruminant and nonruminant?
3. What does the presence of lignin do to cellulose digestion?
4. Why are young plants more readily digestible than older plants?

BIBLIOGRAPHY

Bailey, R., Monro, J., Pickmere, S., and Chesson, A. 1976. Herbage hemicellulose and its digestion by the ruminant. *In* Carbohydrate Research in Plants and Animals. H. Veenman & Zonen B. V., Wagenigen, The Netherlands.
Baumgardt, B. 1969. Utilization of cellulose by ruminants. *In* Cellulases and Their Application. G. S. Hajny and E. T. Reese (Editors). Adv. Chem. Ser. 95, pp. 242–244. Am. Chem. Soc., Washington, D.C.
Church, D. (Editor). 1979. Digestive Physiology and Nutrition of Ruminants, Vol. 2. O and B Books, Corvallis, Oregon.
Crawford, R. 1981. Lignin Biodegradation and Transformation. John Wiley & Sons, New York.
Gray, G. 1970. Carbohydrate digestion and absorption. Gasteroenterology *58*, 96–107.
MacAllister, R. 1979. Nutritive sweeteners made from starch. Adv. Carbohydr. Chem. Biochem. *36*, 15–56.
Pigden, W., and Heaney, D. 1969. Lignocellulose in ruminant nutrition. *In* Cellulases and Their Applications. G. J. Hajny and E. T. Reese (Editors). Adv. Chem. Ser. 95, pp. 245–261. Am. Chem. Soc., Washington, D.C.
Ruckebusch, Y., and Thivend, P. 1980. Digestive Physiology and Metabolism in Ruminants. AVI Publishing Co., Westport, Connecticut.
Wolin, M. 1981. Fermentation in the rumen and human large intestine. Science *213*, 1463–1468.
Yan, J. 1982. Kinetics of delignification: a molecular approach. Science *215*, 1390–1392.

6

High Fiber Diets

A. TYPES OF DIETARY FIBER

The amount of fiber in Western diets has changed considerably in the last century. Not only has the percentage of fiber in the diet dropped from 8 to 3% but the distribution has changed as well with drastic drops in fiber from cereal, potatoes, and legumes especially (Scala 1975). Based largely on epidemiological data, there has been increasing concern that diets low in fiber contribute to the etiology or severity of such diseases as diabetes, hypercholesterolemia, diverticular disease, colonic cancer, obesity, and hemorrhoids. Studies have been undertaken to asses the role of fiber in these diseases and to determine the mechanism(s) whereby fiber might act.

Dietary fiber is plant material resistant to digestion by secretions of the human *small intestine. Crude fiber,* a far less useful term, is the material left after digestion with hot acid and hot alkali. Dietary fiber is 2–6 times the crude fiber content of food. It should not be supposed, however, that dietary fiber is totally indigestible. Although it is not digested in the small intestine (by definition), it may be patially digested and fermented in the colon by colon microflora to yield volatile fatty acids. Some animals, such as rabbits, may even derive a considerable portion of their energy from the fermentation products produced by the colon microflora.

The degree of digestibility of dietary fiber is proportional to its composition. Although cellulose and some of the hemicelluloses may be partially digestible, the degree to which they are accessible to the microflora depends to a large extent on the degree of lignification. Material with high levels of lignin is not very digestible because the lignin acts as a physical barrier between the cellulose or hemicellulose and the microflora. As the age of the plant increases so does the lignin content. Thus, tender young lettuse is more digestible than old tree branches.

B. FIBER AND DIABETES

One of the proposed benefits of dietary fiber is on glucose tolerance in diabetics. Studies have been done with humans using a variety of different dietary regimens to which various types of fiber have been added. In a study evaluating guar, pectin, gum tragacanth, methyl-cellulose, wheat bran, or the drug cholestyramine for effectiveness in decreasing glucose and insulin levels after a 50 g glucose tolerance test, it was found that guar was the most effective (Jenkins *et al.* 1978). However, there seems to be some disparity concerning the effects of fiber on different groups of diabetics. It has been reported that diabetics with neuropathy benefited less from addition of fiber to their diets than did diabetics without neuropathy (Levitt *et al.* 1980). This may be due to the impaired motility of gut in diabetics with neuropathy. Thus, the effect of fiber in decreasing transit time of material through the gut can only work if intestinal motility is not impaired because of nerve damage.

The effect of fiber on dietary lipid absorption has also been of interest. Pectin, especially, has been useful in lowering serum and liver cholesterol levels and in elevating fecal sterol excretin. Pectin, which contains a high percentage of anhydrogalacturonic acid, is found in many fruits and vegetables and is added to jellies to aid in the setting process. The effect of pectin on sterol levels is not restricted to humans but also has been reported for pigs and poultry (Chenoweth and Leveille 1975). The galactomannans (guar gum) and carrageenan have been reported to be even more effective than pectin in lowering serum cholesterol (Stancioff and Renn 1966). When the fiber is fed as unpurified plant material some of the cholesterol lowering effect may be the result of plant sitosterols inhibiting endogenous cholesterol synthesis.

C. MECHANISMS OF FIBER ACTION

The mechanism(s) by which fiber acts has not been clearly elucidated. There are several hypotheses as to its function which are at least partially supported by the available data. The first of these has to do with the altered transit time of fecal material through the gut. Foods containing insoluble plant fibers move through the gut more quickly. If material passes more rapidly, pushing other dietary components along with it, then perhaps certain dietary components are not absorbed as efficiently if they get moved beyond the sites of their maximum absorption.

In addition, if toxic products are formed as the result of microbial or digestive action on dietary constituents, these products would not be in the gut as long if transit time is decreased. Thus, the toxins would not have sufficient time to interact with gut cells to promote colonic cancer, assuming, of course, that this is a valid mechanism for induction of colonic cancer.

Although there is some increased loss of nutrients by the fecal elimination route when high fiber diets are fed, the increase is not dramatic. Another potential effect of dietary fiber is that fiber supplies some unknown micronutrient. If different fibers had differing concentrations of this micronutrient, one could account for the variability of effects due to the type of fiber. To date, however, a fiber contaminant whose concentration correlates well with fiber effects has not been found.

Another feasible mechanism is that fiber interacts with gut cells to release some gut hormone. A prime candidate has been gastric inhibitory polypeptide (GIP), which is known to be involved in the enteroinsular axis and thus would presumably alter glucose tolerance. There is little evidence, however, that this is the case. There may be interactions with other gut hormones, but these possibilities have not been investigated.

Fibers may actually have several modes of action. The more soluble fibers absorb large quantities of water and could potentially form gel filtration columns in the gut. Thus, nutrients could actually be "chromatographed" during intestinal passage. Since fiber gels are all cation binders, there is a possibility that some other nutrients (minerals, vitamins) may be depleted initially, but this does not seem to be a problem with long-term supplementation with dietary fiber (Jenkins et al. 1978).

Available evidence suggests that inclusion of indigestible carbohydrate in the form of fiber in dietary regimens is a beneficial practice. It is particularly helpful for patients with diverticulitis, hemorrhoids, and other maladies of the large intestine. The stool size becomes markedly larger and softer so there is less damage to the tract due to straining to pass the material. There may be added benefits from the lower amount of time that fecal material is in contact with the cells of the gastrointestinal tract. A great deal must be learned about the role of fiber in the digestive process, however, before any definitive statements about mode of action or mechanisms of any ultimate effects can be made.

D. SUMMARY

Dietary fiber is defined as material resistant to digestion by secretions of the human small intestine. In contrast, crude fiber, however, is what is left over after digestion with hot acid and hot alkali. Digestion and fermentation can occur in the large intestine, which in some species may provide a significant number of calories to the animal. Inclusion of fiber in the diet is said to be effective in improving glucose tolerance in diabetics, reducing serum cholesterol, and preventing hemorrhoids and other diseases of the bowel. The mechanisms of action of fiber have not been clearly delineated. There are, however, several possibilities for the effects of fiber including a decrease in transit time. This would have the effect of "washing out" material from the gut thereby reducing nutrient absorbtion and shortening the time that harmful materials are in contact with the gut lining. Fiber could contain some as yet unidentified micronutrient or it could interact with gut hormones to trigger the subsequent observed physiological phenomena.

REVIEW QUESTIONS

1. What is the difference between dietary fiber and crude fiber?
2. What are three possible mechanisms of action of dietary fiber?
3. What does fiber do to fecal sterol concentrations? Serum cholesterol concentrations?

BIBLIOGRAPHY

Anderson, J., Midgley, W., and Wedman, B.   1979.   Fiber and diabetes. Diabetes Care 2, 369–379.
Chenoweth, W., and Leveille, G.   1975.   Metabolism and physiological effects of pectins. In Physiological Effects of Food Carbohydrates. A. Jeanes and J. Hodge (Editors). ACS Symp. Ser. 15. Am. Chem. Soc., Washington, D.C.
Jenkins, D., Wolever, T., Leeds, A., Gassull, M., Haismann, P., Dilawari, D., Goff, D., Metz, G., and Alberti, K.   1978. Dietary fibers, fiber analogues and glucose tolerance: importance of viscosity. Brit. Med. J. 1, 1392–1394.
Jenkins, D., Wolever, T., Nineham, R., Taylor, R., Metz, G., Bacon, S., and Hockaday, T.   1978.   Guar crispbread in the diabetic diet. Brit. Med. J. 2, 1744–1746.
Kay, R., and Strasberg, S.   1978.   Origin, chemistry, physiological effects and clinical importance of dietary fiber. Clin. Invest. Med. 1, 9–24.
Levitt, N., Vinik, A., Sive, A., Child, P., and Jackson, W.   1980.   The effect of dietary fiber on glucose and hormone responses to a mixed meal in normal subjects and in diabetic subjects with and without autonomic neuropathy. Diabetes Care 3, 515–519.
Palumbo, P., Briones, E., and Nelson, R.   1978.   High fiber diet in hyperlipemia. J. Am. Med. Assoc. 240, 223–227.
Scala, J.   1975.   The physiological effects of dietary fiber. In physiological Effects of Food Carbohydrates. A. Jeanes and J. Hodge (Editors). ACS Symp. Ser. 15. Am. Chem. Soc., Washington, D.C.
Stanicioff, D., and Renn, D. 1975. Physiological effects of carrageenan. In Physiological Effects of Food Carbohydrates. A. Jeanes and J. Hodge (Editors). ACS Symp. Ser. 15. Am. Chem. Soc., Washington, D.C.

7

Relationship of Digestive Processes to Regulation of Metabolic Events

A number of events related to the digestive process per se help to regulate subsequent metabolic processes in the body. In effect, there is a "prepriming" of the body for nutrients it will receive as the result of the digestion of food in the gastrointestinal (GI) tract. The advantage to the animal is that the prepriming provides for homeostatic control of the nutrient pools entering the body, thus avoiding wide swings in the blood levels of such nutrients as glucose and amino acids. Further, satiety and selective desires for particular nutrients may also be controlled. Certainly, the rate of passage of the contents of the gut through the tract, which ultimately controls the amount of nutrients absorbed through the mucosal cells, is regulated.

Most of the communication between the GI tract and the rest of the body is carried out either by gut hormones or by nerve impulses. Regulation of insulin levels, satiety, and the rate of transit of material in the gut are most likely all regulated to a significant degree by gut hormones which are secreted by specific cells at various parts of the GI tract. These enter into the general circulation and eventually arrive at their target tissues where they exert their effects. Some may act in a more restrictive fashion by being "local hormones," which cause some action at a cell in close proximity to the secretory cell. These local hormones usually have very short half-lives and are found in very low concentrations in the general circulation. This chapter includes a discussion of some of the actions of gut hormones and their roles in the communication between the GI tract and the rest of the body. The functions of these gut hormones are summarized in Table 7.1.

A. ENTEROINSULAR AXIS AND GASTRIC INHIBITORY POLYPEPTIDE

It has long been known that oral glucose elevates serum insulin to a greater extent than does glucose infused intravenously (i.v.) to give the

TABLE 7.1. Properties of Some Putative Gut Hormones

Hormone	No. amino acids	Actions
Gastric inhibitory polypeptide	43	Insulin release
Cholecystokinin	33	Gallbladder contraction and pancreatic enzyme secretion
Gastrin	17 or 34	Stomach HCl production
Secretin	27	Pancreatic H_2O and bicarbonate secretion
Motilin	22	Upper tract motility
Vasoactive intestinal peptide	28	Gut contractility
Substance P	11	Gut contractility
Neurotensin	13	Ileal contractions and insulin release
Somatostatin	14 (cyclic)	Release inhibiting hormone
Pancreatic polypeptide	34	Alters avian carbohydrate and lipid metabolism
Coherin	32	Jejunal contraction
Urogastrone	52	Gastric acid secretion

same blood glucose values as oral glucose. The eating of a nutrient is, therefore, not necessarily equivalent to receiving the same nutrient by a nonoral route. It has been proposed that there is some effect of glucose on the gut which alters insulin release. This glucose effect on insulin has come to be known as the enteroinsular axis. For some time efforts were made to find a compound that is released by the gut in response to oral dietary intake. This compound would then act on the β cell of the pancreas in such a way as to enhance insulin release.

The best candidate for this action so far is the putative gut hormone *gastric inhibitory polypeptide* (GIP) sometimes referred to as glucose-dependent insulin-releasing polypeptide to be more descriptive of its physiological action. It may well not be the only hormone involved in the enteroinsular axis.

GIP was discovered in 1969 by Brown and his colleagues in cholecystokinin–pancreozymin extracts. This peptide is 43 amino acids long with a molecular weight of approximately 5100. It is found in cells in the duodenal region and to a lesser extent in the jejunal region of the gut. The amino acid sequence of 15 of the first 26 amino acids on the N terminal end are identical with the homone porcine glucagon and 9 are the same as secretin but the 17 amino acids on the C-terminal end are unique with respect to other gut hormones. The active portion of the molecule would presumably be in this C-terminal region of the protein. In addition to its effect on insulin release it inhibits gastrin-, pentagastrin-, insulin-, and histamine-stimulated gastric acid secretion.

GIP is released biphasically, first in response to dietary carbohydrate, then in response to fat. The released GIP then migrates to the pancreas via the bloodstream. If glucose is present, GIP promotes release of insulin from the β cell. In the absence of glucose GIP has no effect. The details of insulin release are discussed in Chapter 11. The role of GIP in diabetes has been of considerable concern. Lowered response of the β cells to GIP has been noted in obese and non-insulin-dependent diabetics. There is an elevated secretion of GIP but a lowered output of insulin at the same time. Some types of impaired glucose tolerance or diabetes could be the result of an impairment of regulation at the level of gut hormones.

B. OTHER GUT HORMONES IMPORTANT IN DIGESTIVE REGULATION

It is apparent that a number of gut hormones other than GIP are important in overall digestive regulation as well. Although these hormones may not play as direct a role as GIP in carbohydrate metabolism, they are important in the overall digestive process. Not only are the various digestive processes within the tract regulated but there is also regulation and communication of what is happening in the gut with the rest of the body. Gastric acid secretion, motility, zymogen secretion, control of small intestine pH, and satiety are all under the apparent control of gut hormones.

The components of the digestive tracts of three representative species are given in Table 7.2. Humans and other nonruminant mammals have digestive tracts very similar to that of the pig. Even the digestive systems of avian species and ruminants are not really so very different than nonruminants as it might seem at first glance. The hormones and enzymes secreted, the locations where these are found, and their modes of action are really remarkably similar. Granted, a ruminant GI tract

TABLE 7.2. Components of the Gastrointestinal Tracts from Mouth to Anus of Three Species

Pig	Chicken	Cow
Mouth	Mouth	Mouth
Esophagus	Esophagus	Esophagus
Stomach	Crop	Reticulum
Duodenum	Proventriculus	Abomasum
Jejunum	Duodenum	Omasum
Ileum	Gizzard	Rumen
Caecum	Jejunum	Duodenum
Colon	Ileum	Jejunum
Rectum	Caecum	Ileum
Anus	Rectum	Caecum
	Cloaca	Colon
		Rectum
		Anus

has a few extra compartments, but these are in addition to, rather than instead of, what occurs in the nonruminant.

In order to assume hormonal status, a compound must meet the following criteria: (1) secretion in one part of the tract must result in a response in a distant target; (2) effects must persist after neural connections are severed; (3) the event must be mimicked by an injection of an extract of the stimulated part but no other parts; (4) the amount and kind of peptide released must be correlated with the event; and (5) the event must be able to be copied in *in vitro* experiments. Hormonal status is generally accorded to the following gut hormones even though all these criteria have not been met: gastrin, secretin, cholecystokinin–pacreozymin, pancreatic polypeptide, gastric inhibitory polypeptide, motilin, vasoactive intestinal polypeptide, and enteroglucagon. A number of other gut peptides have been chemically characterized but their functions are less certain. There are also a number of events in the gut which are clearly hormonally controlled, but these events have not yet been associated with a hormone.

There may need to be some revision in our thinking regarding "gut hormones." First, gut hormones do not occur exclusively in the gut. Substance P, somatostatin, cholecystokinin–pancreozymin, vasoactive intestinal polypeptide, enkephalin, bombesin, and neurotensin all are found in the central nervous system as well. They may function as *circulating hormones, local hormones,* or *neurotransmitters* in the autonomic nervous system. It has been suggested (Polak and Bloom 1978) that a third class of neuron be added to the two presently recognized types (adrenergic and cholinergic). This type would be called "peptidergic" and is derived embryologically from the neuroendocrine programmed ectoblast. Thus, some of the gut hormones seem to be derived from two types of cells: the neuroendocrine cells and true endocrine cells derived from epithelial cells. This challenges one of the classical criteria for a hormone, that is, that a hormone is found in an epithelial-type cell and anything originating from a neuroendocrine cell is a neuroendocrine effector.

The second challenge to our traditional thinking concerns the number of hormones per cell. In the past, it has been tacitly assumed that there is one hormone per cell. Substance P and serotonin are, however, both found in the same cells and there are other cases of this duality as well.

One of the most important gut hormones is *cholecystokinin.* This hormone is also referred to as pancreozymin. Ivy and Oldberg in 1928 found a peptide that activated gallbladder contractions, and then in 1943 Harper and Raper found a compound which stimulated pancreatic enzyme secretion (for a review see Rayford *et al.* 1976). They named it pancreozymin. Still later it became clear that these two were one in the same compound. Although the recommended name is cholecystokinin it is still often referred to as the hyphenated version of the two names or as the abbreviation CCK-PZ.

Cholecystokinin is found both in the gut and in the brain. It contains 33 amino acids. The eight C-terminal amino acids are the important, reactive portion of this molecule; in fact this section has greater activity than the parent molecule. Cholecystokinin also has a sulfated tyrosine, but it is not presently known whether sulfation/desulfation could be a covalent modification controlling the potency of the hormone. Cholecystokinin is rapidly cleared from the circulation by the kidney.

It stimulates gallbladder contraction and pancreatic enzyme secretion. Its release from cells in the duodenum and upper intestine is promoted by amino acids, fatty acids, HCl, and the process of eating. Perhaps one of its most important functions is in the promotion of satiety. It has been found (Straus and Yalow 1979) that its concentration in the brains of genetically obese (ob/ob) mice is an order of magnitude lower than in the brains of lean controls. Since the hypothalamus is thought to control satiety, it is not difficult to propose a mechanism for how satiety signals could be accomplished. For example, chewing a candy bar promotes salivation, which in turn solubilizes sugar. The sugar binds to the lectins on the taste buds eliciting a nerve impulse, which is sent to the brain. The nerve impulse triggers the release of cholecystokinin, which migrates to the hypothalamus, signaling satiety and shutting off feeding behavior. Though this is pure conjecture, such a mechanism is surely attractive. It has been shown that cerebroventricular injections of cholecystokinin promote satiety in sheep (Della-Fera and Baile 1979). If such a mechanism is valid, the implications for those of us who gulp our food are clear. An important regulatory mechanism for control of feeding is bypassed, and an excessive amount of food is consumed before satiety is reached.

Another very important hormone is gastrin. It was discovered in 1905 and is found in the G cells of the pylorus and pancreas. The function of gastrin is to stimulate HCl secretion in the stomach. In high concentrations, it causes trophic effects on mucosal cells. In Zollinger–Ellison syndrome there is a pancreatic islet cell tumor with many small foci. This tumor promotes high levels of gastrin to be released from the pancreas causing excess acid production and massive stomach ulceration. Since it is usually not possible to remove the tumors from the pancreas, the target tissue, the stomach, is removed instead. This syndrome is usually not fatal and one can live without a stomach.

Gastrin was originally isolated by Gregory and Tracy (Thompson 1975) from 50,000 hog antrums. It occurs in several molecular forms which have different half-lives: G-17, a 17 amino acid species, G-34, the predominant species in the intestine, and big-big gastrin, the principal circulating species. Big-big gastrin is probably gastrin attached to some of the large circulating proteins. G-17 exists in two forms depending on whether or not the tyrosine is sulfated. Gastrin II is the sulfated form and gastrin I is unsulfated. The five C-terminal amino acids compose the reactive portion of the molecule. This fragment is called *pentagastrin,* and many of the studies done on gastrin have employed this fragment. Gastrin is eliminated from the body primarily by the kidney and secondarily by the liver.

Secretin is another hormone important to the overall digestive process. It was the first hormone discovered. It is secreted by the S cells of the duodenum in response to H^+ washing over this area. Secretin stimulates the secretion of water and bicarbonate from the pancreas as a result. This has the effect of raising the pH in the upper small intestine so that the hydrolytic enzymes, which usually have pH optima of between 5 and 7, can function. Secretin is a very basic, 27 amino acid peptide containing four arginines, one histidine, and having two of the three glutamates amidated in the γ-carboxyl. Unlike cholecystokinin or gastrin, which have active fragments, the entire secretin molecule is required for activity. Secretin is rapidly inactivated by liver with a $t_{1/2}$ of only 2.5 min.

There are a number of other gut peptides of less certain status. Among these are motilin, vasoactive intestinal peptide, neurotesin, substance P, and enteroglucagon. There are also some nongut hormones with potent effects on the gut. These include pancreatic polypeptide, somatostatin coherin, and urogasterone. The information available about these putative hormones is summarized below.

Motlin is a 22 amino acid peptide released from the enterochromaffin cells of the small intestine by alkalization of the duodenum. Motilin stimulates the motile activity of the upper tract. There is a marked species difference in the concentration of this hormone; it is high in man.

Vasoactive intestinal polypeptide (VIP), a 28 amino acid peptide, is found in highest concentration in the small intestine but is widely scattered along the length of the G.I. tract in both mammalian and avian species. It is a potent vasodilator, but it also has a number of effects on the gasterointestinal tract. It relaxes isolated tracheas from guinea pigs, inhibits acid secretion stimulated by histamine or pentagastrin, inhibits pepsin secretion while stimulating pancreatic secretion and biliary secretion, and enhances gut contractility. VIP is inactivated predominantly by the liver. Its very rapid turnover suggests it may be a local hormone. It is found in high concentrations in individuals with Verner–Morrison syndrome. In this disease tumors cause release of large quantities of VIP and extreme watery diarrhea is the result.

Substance P is a hypotensive and gut contractile agent. It was initially derived from powdered extracts of the intestine and hence the P stands for powder. It is rather smaller than other gut hormones being only 11 amino acids long. It is found associated with serotonin in cells and is high in patients with carcinoid tumors.

Neurotensin is derived from N cells and is a 13 amino acid peptide. It stimulates ileal contractions and inhibits insulin release. In coeliac disease, a diabetic-like syndrome arises. There is an enteropathy of the gut such that gastrin release is normal, gastric inhibitory polypeptide and secretin are greatly reduced, and neurotensin and enteroglucagon are elevated. In effect, insulin release stimulation is abolished and inhibition of insulin release is favored resulting in a typical diabetes-like syndrome because neurotensin is a potent inhibitor of insulin release.

Enteroglucagon cross reactions in antibody reactions with true glucagon but it is likely to have a different physiological role. It is produced in L cells of the lower jejunum and colon. This peptide has been difficult to characterize because of the cross-reactivity, but there appear to be two peaks of activity on molecular sieve chromatography, one of which has about twice the molecular weight of the other. Both fractions are present in about equal concentrations in the gut and in circulation. The concentration of enteroglucagon is elevated when glucose and other monosaccharides are being absorbed. When dogs are surgically altered such that they can no longer produce enterogucagon there is a large accumulation of liver glycogen. It may be that entero-glucagon regulates the upper extent to which glycogen can be synthesized and stored.

Of the nongut hormones with potent effects, *somatostatin* seems to play a general role. It is a 14 amino acid, cyclic peptide secreted by the D cells of the pancreas and also found in the hypothalamus. Somato-statin is a release inhibiting hormone. That is, it prevents the release of a number of hormones such as insulin, glucagon, growth hormone, and all the known gut hormones. In a physiological situation, it proba-bly acts locally because its general release would be expected to shut down release of all peptide hormones indiscriminately.

Pancreatic polypeptide, a linear, 36 amino acid peptide, is found in high concentration in some tumors. It affects carbohydrate and lipid metabolism in birds. Although it rises in response to food in the gut, it does not seem to be directly related to specific dietary components.

Coherin has 32 amino acids, comes from the neurohypophysis, and stimulates jejunal contractions. *Urogastrone* is 52 amino acids long and appears in urine. It inhibits gastric acid secretion. Relatively little is known about these two peptides.

The gut hormones fall into families of hormones based on shared amino acid sequence. One such family is the secretin–glucagon family whose members are secretin, glucagon, VIP, and GIP. Fourteen amino acid residues share the same positions in glucagon and in secretin. This may imply that they have arisen from a similar parent molecule over the course of evolutionary time. It is clear that quite a number of peptides are likely involved in the digestive process itself and in pre-priming the body for the arrival of nutrients. The gut hormones briefly discussed here by no means comprise the complete list of known hor-mones. Even though the list is large, it is probable that it will undergo expansion over the next few years. The reader is referred to further information about these additional compounds in several of the excellent review articles listed in the Bibliography at the end of this chapter.

C. SUMMARY

The enteroinsular axis describes the effect of food in the gut on the release of insulin from the pancreas. Insulin release is greater from oral glucose than from glucose given i.v., an effect thought to be due to the action of the gut hormone gastric inhibitory polypeptide. Other putative gut hormones are involved in the digestive process as well. Their functions include stimulation of stomach acid secretion (gastrin), pancreatic enzyme secretion (cholecystokinin), and water and bicarbonate secretion (secretin). Several hormones alter the contractility of various portions of the tract. These include motilin, VIP, substance P, neurotensin, and coherin. These may have other actions as well. Somatostatin is somewhat unique in that it is a cyclic peptide and is capable of inhibiting the release of a number of other hormones. Research in the area of gut hormones is really just beginning, and great progress may be expected in the next decade.

REVIEW QUESTIONS

1. What gut hormone is presently most implicated in the enteroinsular axis?
2. What two hormones contribute to pancreatic secretion of enzymes and bicarbonate?
3. What hormone inhibits the release of numerous other hormones?
4. Which hormones seem to be involved in gastrointestinal tract motility?

BIBLIOGRAPHY

Brown, J., Pederson, R., and Jorpes, E. 1969. Preparation of a highly active entero-
    gastrone. Can. J. Physiol. Pharmacol. 47, 113–114.
Brown, J., Dahl, M., Kwarik, S., McIntosh, C., Otte, S., and Pederson, R. 1981. Actions
    of GIP. Peptides 2, Suppl. 2, 241–246.
Bueno, L., and Ferre, J.-P. 1982. Central regulation of intestinal motility by
    somatostatin and cholecystokinin octapeptide. Science 216, 1427–1429.
Della-Fera, M., and Baile, C. 1979. Cholecystokinin octapeptide: continuous picomole
    injections into the cerebral ventricles of sheep supress feeding. Science 206,
    471–473.
Erspamer, V., Melchiorri, P. Broccardo, M., Erspamer, G., Falaschi, P., Improta, G.,
    Negri, L., and Renda, T. 1981. The brain-gut-skin triangle: new peptides. Pep-
    tides 2 Suppl. 2, 7–16.
Grossman, M. 1974. Candidate hormones of the gut. Gasteroenterology 67, 730–755.
Gullner, H. 1982. Gastrin releasing peptide. IRCS Med. Sci. Biochem. 10, 450–451.
Johnson, L. 1979. Comparative biochemistry and physiology of gut hormones. Annu.
    Rev. Physiol. 39, 135–158.
Morley, J. 1982. The ascent of cholecystokinin from gut to brain. Life Sci. 30,
    479–494.

Polak, J., and Bloom, S. 1978. Peptidergic innervation of the gasterointestinal tract. Adv. Expl. Med. Biol. *106*, 27–49.

Rayford, P., Miller, T., and Thompson, J. 1976. Secretin, Cholecystokinin and newer gasterointestinal hormones. New Eng. J. Med. *294*, 1093–1101, 1157–1164.

Straus, E., and Yalow, R. 1979. Cholecystokinin in the brains of obese and nonobese mice. Science *203*, 68–69.

Thompson, J. (Editor). 1975. Gastrointestinal Hormones: A Symposium. Univ. of Texas Press, Austin, Texas.

Part III

Carbohydrate Metabolism

8

The Metabolic Fate of Glucose

A. TISSUE DISTRIBUTION

Glucose is not an obligatory dietary nutrient for any higher animals. It does, however, play a number of very important biochemical roles in every species. It is the preferred fuel for the central nervous system. If blood glucose levels drop too low, the functioning of the central nervous system becomes impaired. The body has several mechanisms (gluconeogenesis and glycogenolysis) whereby glucose can be supplied to the bloodstream when it is not available from the diet. Glucose also serves as a precursor for a number of cellular constituents such as glycogen, fat, nonessential amino acids, other sugars, and the ribose moiety of nucleic acids or it can be oxidized to CO_2 and H_2O for energy (Fig. 8.1).

We will first consider the fate of dietary glucose available as the result of the ingestion of glucose per se, or of starch, glycogen, sucrose, or lactose. After being actively transported across the gut wall, glucose enters the portal circulation and to a large measure is removed by the liver. During the fed state, blood glucose levels will be elevated as will insulin levels, and the liver will effectively trap much of the glucose arriving from the portal circulation by phosphorylating the glucose to

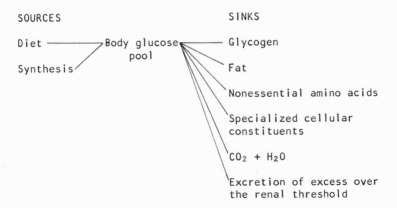

FIG. 8.1. Sources and sinks for glucose in the body.

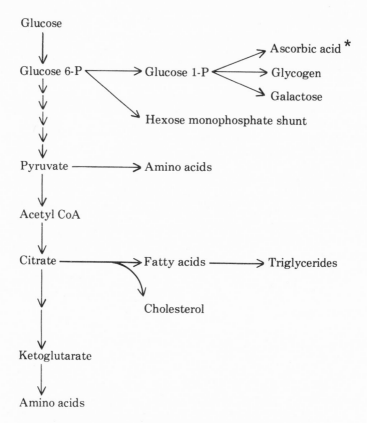

FIG. 8.2. Intracellular utilization of glucose. *Except for primates, guinea pigs, and the Indian fruit bat.

glucose 6-phosphate. Since phosphorylated compounds do not cross intact cell membranes, glucose is filtered out of the circulation in this manner. Glucose enters the liver cells on a specific carrier. How much glucose is taken up by the liver depends on the blood glucose concentration and the hormonal status of the animal. Although insulin is not needed for glucose entry into liver cells, high insulin levels are conducive to glucose utilization by the liver because of the effect of insulin on subsequent enzymatic steps.

Other tissues also compete for available blood glucose. The central nervous system, of course, has the edge since uptake into this tissue is dependent neither on blood glucose levels nor on insulin concentrations. Tissues such as muscle and adipose cells can only remove glucose from the bloodstream with the aid of insulin. This ensures that such tissues, which can easily use other substrates, will rely on glucose only when there is an abundant supply, that is, in the fed state when carbohydrate is available from the diet and insulin levels are high.

Besides obtaining glucose from the diet, there are only two tissues that can supply glucose to the bloodstream: liver and kidney. These are the only organs able to carry out gluconeogenesis from lactate or amino acids. In addition they can, of course, break down glycogen to serve as a source of blood glucose as well. Although muscle and adipose tissue have stores of glycogen, these stores can only be broken down for use in these locations because these tissues lack glucose-6-phosphatase which is necessary to dephosphorylate the glucose 6-phosphate so that glucose can escape into the bloodstream.

Once glucose has been taken up by an organ (e.g., liver), what determines which pathway receives the glucose? It depends on the relative rates of the enzymes in the possible pathways. Figure 8.2 shows some of the options for glucose. For a review, each separate pathway will be briefly discussed below. It has been proposed (Ureta 1978) that multi-enzyme complexes may exist and that the end product may be a function of which pathway a substrate entered. Therefore, the pathway selected might be a function of which enzyme in the various pathways was able to act on the substrate initially.

B. GLYCOLYSIS

The glycolytic pathway is shown in Fig. 8.3. The principal control points are at the hexokinase/glucokinase, the phosphofructokinase, and the pyruvate kinase steps. As an energy producing pathway, glycolysis yields only a net of two ATPs produced per glucose molecule. If one views lactate as the end product of the pathway, it can be seen that lactate and glucose have the same oxidation state. The energy recovered by this pathway, therefore, reflects only the breaking of the bond between C-3 and C-4, and no oxidation of glucose has occurred to this point. Oxidative phosphorylation, on the other hand, provides a great deal more energy because the remaining C—C bonds are broken and the carbons become fully oxidized to CO_2. Some cells, such as mature red blood cells, nonetheless must rely on glycolysis as their energy source because they lack mitochondria and therefore the capacity to carry out oxidative phosphorylation. For a red blood cell, however, this is not a serious problem because this cell needs little energy for synthetic reactions or for contractile events. The bulk of its energy requirement is probably spent keeping K^+ inside the cell and Na^+ outside the cell. Cancer cells likewise rely heavily on glycolysis for their energy demands.

The first step in glycolysis is the phosphorylation of glucose which results in trapping of glucose inside a cell. This step is catalyzed by one of the *hexokinases*. Most of the forms of hexokinase (Types I, II, and III) have low K_m's for glucose (10^{-5}–10^{-7} M), all of which are little effected by diet. Type IV hexokinase, however, has a K_m for glucose of 10^{-2} M and is found essentially only in the parenchymal cells of the

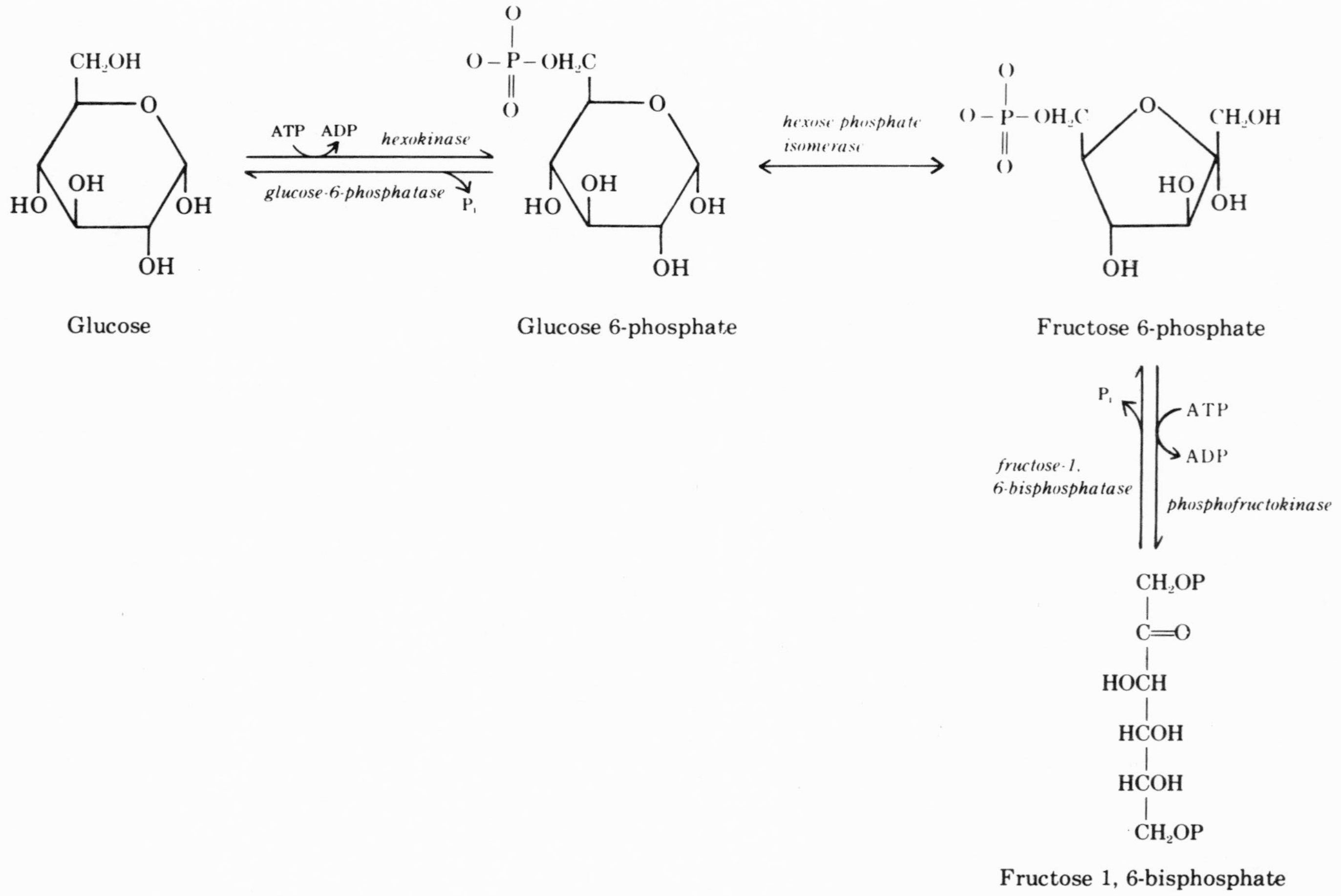

CH₂OH

OH

HO

OH

O

Glucose

ATP ADP

hexokinase

glucose-6-phosphatase

Pᵢ

O

O—P—OH₂C

O

OH

OH

HO

OH

O

Glucose 6-phosphate

hexose phosphate isomerase

CH₂OH

OH

HO

OH

O

O

O—P—OH₂C

O

Fructose 6-phosphate

Pᵢ

ATP

ADP

fructose-1, 6-bisphosphatase

phosphofructokinase

CH₂OP

C=O

HOCH

HCOH

HCOH

CH₂OP

Fructose 1, 6-bisphosphate

64

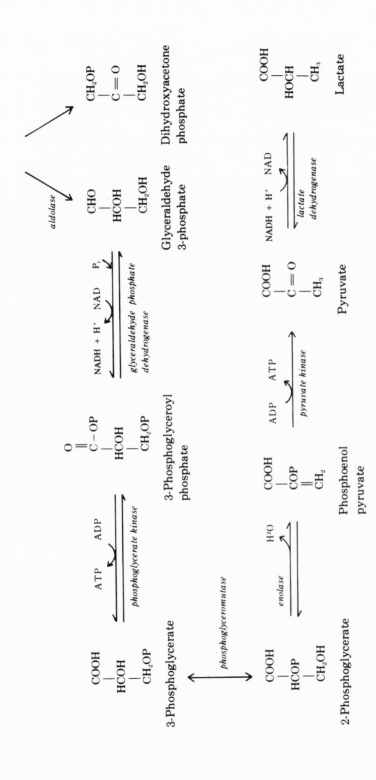

FIG. 8.3.   Glycolysis.

liver under conditions of high dietary glucose and high insulin. The activity of this type of hexokinase follows a circadian rhythm related to food intake. It is called *glucokinase* and is present in the livers of those animals which one would expect to encounter high dietary glucose, i.e., mice, rats, guinea pigs, rabbits, dogs, pigs, and man, and is low or absent in livers of animals who have low circulating glucose levels (cats and ruminant species such as cows, sheep, quokkas, and tamars). Diabetics also have low glucokinase activity, and it is also absent, as one would suppose, in fetal liver.

Usually the hexokinases are found in the soluble (cytoplasmic) portion of the cell. Type I is found predominately in brain and Type II is usually found in muscle cells. Their activities are inhibited to varying extents by the product of the reaction, glucose 6-phosphate. A rather interesting phenomenon occurs in the case of brain hexokinase Type I. If chickens are made to become ischemic and the oxygen supply to the brain is impaired, hexokinase migrates from the cytoplasm and attaches itself to the outside of the mitochondria. As the result of this apparent change in compartments, the inhibition by glucose 6-phosphate is markedly reduced and the K_m for ATP drops fivefold from 1.7 to 0.34 μM. In effect, this sustains the ability of the brain to function for an additional period. Even though oxidative phosphorylation is impaired due to lack of oxygen resulting in a loss of the major source of ATP generation, glycolysis can still function and provide small amounts of ATP. The shift in K_m's and inhibition characteristics ensures that glycolysis has an opportunity to occur. Enzymes that change characteristics by changing compartments are called *ambiquitous enzymes*.

After glucose is phosphorylated to glucose 6-phosphate (G-6-P), there are some branch points to other pathways. G-6-P may continue in the glycolytic pathway or it may enter the hexose–monophosphate shunt, glycogen synthesis or galactose synthesis, or other such pathways as glucuronate synthesis, etc. If it continues in glycolysis, it is isomerized to fructose 6-phosphate by *hexosephosphate isomerase*. This reaction is readily reversible.

The next step, catalyzed by *phosphofructokinase* (PFK), is also a control point in glycolysis. It is an irreversible reaction and fructose 1,6-bisphosphate is the product. This enzyme has a large number of allosteric modulators. It is activated by fructose 6-phosphate, adenosine monophosphate (AMP), adenosine diphosphate (ADP), and fructose 1,6-bisphosphate. It is inhibited by citrate, ATP, oxygen, phosphocreatine, and fatty acids. The system is even more complex than it would appear at first glance, however, because the degree to which the inhibitors are effective is somewhat dependent on how much substrate (fructose 6-phosphate) is available. There may also be an enzyme–enzyme interaction between phosphofructokinase and the enzyme catalyzing the reverse reaction, fructose 1,6-bisphosphatase. Another complicating factor is the existence of a dietary dependent small molecule described by Dunaway and Segal (1976). This molecule, which seems to be a three amino acid peptide with a long carbohydrate chain tail, is elevated by diets high in carbohydrate or by insulin and is found in low concentration during starvation and diabetes. Although the *in vivo* function of this effector is still unknown, it protects phosphofructokinase against inactivation *in vitro*.

Phosphofructokinase occurs as two isozymes: L_1 and L_2. The L_2 form, which is the more regulatable, predominates in the parenchymal cells of the liver. The enzyme may also fall into the ambiquitous category in that it has been reported to bind reversibly with erythrocyte membranes whereupon it loses its inhibition by ATP, 2,3-bisphosphoglycerate, and citrate.

The activity of phosphofructokinase in liver is lowered by epinephrine and glucagon and elevated by insulin. This is thought to be due to covalent modification of the enzyme by phosphorylation and dephosphorylation. Recently several investigators have found a new modulator of this system, fructose 2,6-bisphosphate, which is an apparent activator. When the enzyme is phosphorylated it seems to be more sensitive to ATP inhibition, and the affinity of the enzyme for the activation factor is decreased. The tissue content of fructose 2,6-bisphosphate is increased by insulin. The enzyme which degrades this effector, fructose 2,6-bisphosphatase, is stimulated by cyclic AMP and inhibited by the product of the reaction, fructose 6-phosphate.

Phosphofructokinase appears to be the site of the Pasteur effect. When a cell has sufficient oxygen, glycolytic activity is low because energy is more efficiently supplied by oxidative phosphorylation. If oxygen supplies are limited, however, a greater amount of substrate must be committed to glycolysis to supply ATP. Presumably, this effect occurs as the result of oxygen inhibition of phosphofructokinase. This regulatory site may be especially important for diving animals. In the initial stages of the dive, oxygen tension is high, glycolysis is low, and oxidative phosphorylation is high. As the dive progresses, oxygen concentration drops, inhibition of phosphofructokinase is released, and an increasing percentage of the animal's energy comes from glucose.

The next series of steps in the glycolytic sequence are physiologically reversible. After phosphofructokinase comes the cleavage of fructose 1,6-bisphosphate to yield dihydroxyacetone phosphate and glyceraldehyde 3-phosphate, catalyzed by *aldolase*. There are several isozymes of aldolase. Type A is found in muscle, type B mainly in liver, and type C in the brain. These aldolases differ from those found in bacteria and other lower life forms in that a divalent metal ion is not required for activity, and there is a different mechanism of reaction.

The products of this reaction are rapidly equilibrated by *triose phosphate isomerase*. The equilibrium mixture of the two compounds greatly favors dihydroxyacetone phosphate (90% of the equilibrium mixture). Further progress in glycolysis, however, occurs via glyceraldehyde 3-phosphate which is next converted to 3-phosphoglyceroyl phosphate (1,3-bisphosphoglycerate), requiring inorganic phosphate and the conversion of NAD to NADH + H$^+$. *Glyceraldehyde-phosphate dehydrogenase,* which catalyzes this reaction, is a tetramer made of four identical subunits each of which bind one NAD. After binding NAD$^+$, the enzyme binds glyceraldehyde phosphate with the aldehyde group forming a thiohemiacetal link with a sulfyhdryl group on the enzyme. A thioester is formed when a hydrogen is transferred from the substrate to NAD to form NADH. The NADH is then exchanged for a new NAD$^+$ from the reaction mixture. Then there is a transfer of phosphate to the acyl group of the substrate as it detaches from the sulfhydryl group of the enzyme. NAD$^+$ is a metabolic effector of this enzyme.

The next step generates ATP and is catalyzed by *phosphoglycerate kinase.* Phosphoglyceroyl phosphate releases its C-1 phosphate to ADP to form ATP and 3-phosphoglycerate. Like all kinases, this enzyme requires Mg^{2+}. In the next reaction 3-phosphoglycerate becomes 2-phosphoglycerate by the action of *phosphoglyceromutase.* The form of the enzyme found in animal tissues requires Mg^{2+} and 2,3-diphosphoglycerate as an intermediate.

The next step in glycolysis is a dehydration of 2-phosphoglycerate to phosphoenolpyruvate catalyzed by *enolase.* This enzyme is relatively small (85,000 MW) and requires Mg^{2+} or Mn^{2+} for activity. Directly after this comes another ATP generating step. *Pyruvate kinase,* which is the third and last control point in glycolysis, catalyzes the conversion of phosphoenolpyruvate to pyruvate with the generation of a molecule of ATP. The step, like the other control points, is irreversible. Like other kinases, pyruvate kinase requires Mg^{2+} for activity. Again, there are several forms of the enzyme: the L form is found in liver parenchymal cells, the M form is the muscle enzyme, and the A form is found in other tissues. The L form of the enzyme is part of a "feedforward" activation system via activation by fructose 1,6-bisphosphate. This enzyme is inhibited by alanine, ATP, AMP, long chain fatty acids, and citrate. It is now known to undergo cyclic AMP dependent phosphorylation/dephosphorylation. The phosphorylation is not a simple turn on/turn off device, however. At low PEP concentrations the enzyme is inhibited by phosphorylation so in essence phosphorylation elevates the K_m for PEP in the absence of fructose 1,6-bisphosphate. In liver perfused with glucagon, the K_m for PEP rose from 1.6 to 2.5 mM (Engstrom 1978). In chicken liver, pyruvate kinase is found in a complex with the protein kinase.

Once pyruvate is formed there are several pathways it may enter. Pyruvate may be reduced to lactate by lactate dehydrogenase and NADH. It may also undergo transamination to form alanine or it can enter the mitochondria to undergo further oxidation. If pyruvate is reduced to lactate, by *lactate dehydrogenase,* the NADH produced at the glyceraldehydephosphate dehydrogenase step is reoxidized to NAD$^+$. The equilibrium of this reaction favors the production of lactate but the reaction is physiologically reversible. There are five isozymes of lactate dehydrogenase which is the number of permutations that two different subunit chains (M chains or H chains) can be put together as a tetrameric enzyme. At each extreme there are all the same type of chain designated M_4 or H_4. M_4 is the type that predominates in skeletal muscle and H_4 is the type found in heart. These isozymes differ in both the K_m and V_{max} of the reaction. The muscle enzyme has a low K_m for pyruvate and a high V_{max} whereas the heart form has a high K_m for pyruvate and a low V_{max}. This difference reflects the metabolic conditions of these tissues in that the heart relies on aerobic metabolism for its energy whereas skeletal muscle has considerable anaerobic glycolysis occurring. Further, the lactate produced by skeletal muscle diffuses out into the bloodstream and is returned to the liver where it can be reconverted to blood glucose. This muscle lactate to liver to glucose to muscle lactate route is known as the *Cori cycle*.

C. TRICARBOXYLIC ACID CYCLE

The tricarboxylic acid cycle (TCA cycle), also known as the citric acid cycle or Krebs cycle after its discoveror, Sir Hans Krebs, in 1937, leads to the oxidation of two carbon fragments in the form of acetyl-CoA. The acetyl-CoA may originally have come from carbohydrates via glycolysis, from fats via β oxidation, or from the degradation of certain amino acids. The bulk of energy recovery occurs as the result of the oxidation occurring in the TCA cycle. Not only are C—C bonds broken but the compounds entering the cycle become more oxidized as well.

The components of the TCA cycle, which is located in the mitochondrial portion of the cell, are shown in Fig. 8.4. Pyruvate enters the mitochondria on a pyruvate carrier. Once inside the mitochondria there are several pathways it may take. If it is to start through the TCA cycle it first must be acted on by *pyruvate dehydrogenase* (PDH).

This enzyme is an enormously large complex composed of five separate enzyme activities: pyruvate dehydrogenase, dihydrolipoyl dehydrogenase, dihydrolipoyl transacetylase, a regulatory kinase, and a phosphatase. The pyruvate dehydrogenase complex from heart or kidney is composed of a core of approximately 60 molecules of dihydrolipoyl transacetylase surrounded by 20 molecules of pyruvate dehydrogenase, five molecules of dihydrolipoyl dehydrogenase, five kinase molecules, and two to three phosphatase molecules. The overall reaction mechanism is simple enough:

$$\text{pyruvate} + \text{CoASH} + \text{NAD}^+ \rightarrow \text{acetyl-CoA} + \text{CO}_2 + \text{NADH} + \text{H}^+$$

In reality, however, the reaction involves a series of enzymatic steps shown in Fig. 8.5. The first step is catalyzed by *pyruvate dehydrogenase* and involves thiamine pyrophosphate, which is covalently attached to

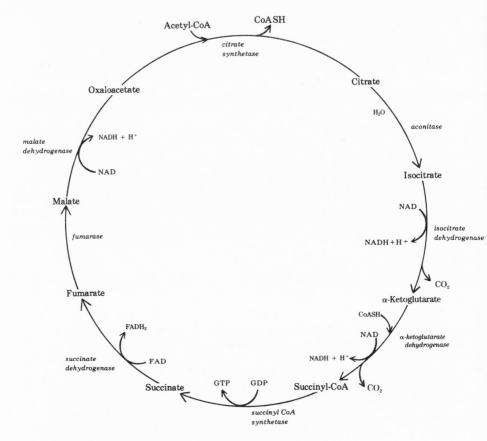

FIG. 8.4.   The tricarboxylic acid (citric acid) cycle.

the pyruvate dehydrogenase moiety. This is the rate-limiting reaction in the sequence.

In this part of the reaction pyruvate is decarboxylated leaving a two carbon α-hydroxyethyl fragment attached to the thiamine pyrophosphate. The second reaction is catalyzed by *dihydrolipoyl transacetylase* which first dehydrogenates the α-hydroxyethyl group then transfers the resultant acetate group to C—6 of the lipoic acid attached to this enzyme and then reacts it with a free CoASH to form acetyl-CoA and the reduced form of lipoate. The final step is needed to return everything to the start. *Dihydrolipoyl dehydrogenase* does this by reoxidizing the lipoate at the expense of enzyme bound FAD. The FADH+ produced is then reconverted to FAD using exogenous NAD+ and converting it to NADH + H+.

The activity of the pyruvate dehydrogenase is high when animals are fed high carbohydrate diets or injected with insulin and low if

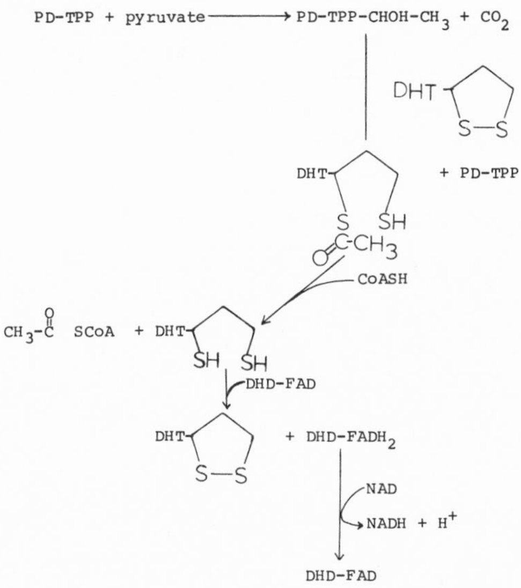

$$\text{PD-TPP} + \text{pyruvate} \longrightarrow \text{PD-TPP-CHOH-CH}_3 + CO_2$$

FIG. 8.5. Pyruvate dehydrogenase reaction mechanism.

animals are fasted or fed high fat low carbohydrate diets. The regulation of the activity of this enzyme is quite as complex as its composition and overall reaction.

The activity of the complex is controlled by a kinase and a phosphatase. The kinase, which is tightly bound to the complex, phosphorylates the pyruvate dehydrogenase component of the complex. This component is an $\alpha_2\beta_2$ tetramer. Phosphorylation occurs on serine residues at three distinct sites (1, 2, and 3) on pyruvate dehydrogenase with the rate being fastest at site 1. Site 1 phosphorylation also correlates well with the activity decline of the complex. The role of the multisite phosphorylations, however, is unclear at the present time.

Dephosphorylation, which activates the enzyme, is catalyzed by a magnesium-dependent phosphatase, which is only loosely associated with the complex. In the presence of calcium, the phosphatase becomes more tightly bound to the complex lowering the K_m of the phosphatase for pyruvate dehydrogenase from 30 to 1.6 μM. It is possible to separate all of the component enzymes without destroying their respective activities, but the overall reaction rate of the individual enzymes is greatly slowed compared to the complex. This is clearly an example of the improvement in kinetics which occurs when a "solid-state" association is formed.

Investigations of the regulation of the kinase and phosphatase have led to some interesting observations. The kinase is not cyclic AMP dependent and does not respond to cyclic AMP directly. In adipose tissue, cyclic AMP is able to block insulin activation of the complex. Further, a small molecule released from cell membranes in response to

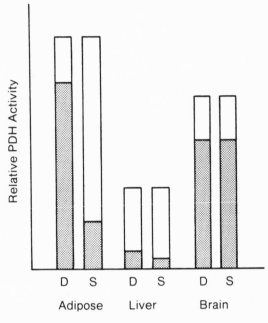

FIG. 8.6. Distribution of active and inactive portions of pyruvate dehydrogenase activity in various tissues from fed and fasted animals. Adapted from Wieland *et al.* (1973). The hatched part of the bars represents the active fraction of PDH activity. D, fed animals; S, fasted animals.

insulin is capable of activating the complex, presumably via activation of the phosphatase. As expected, tissues that are affected by fasting show a marked drop in the active portion of pyruvate dehydrogenase but no changes in total amounts of the enzyme (Fig. 8.6). Further, studies with normal and obese mice indicate (Wieland *et al.* 1973) that although the total activities are similar, there was a higher percentage of active enzyme in the obese mice and their ability to activate the enzyme was also greater.

A number of factors influence the proportion of active to inactive enzyme. Originally, it was believed that these factors were direct metabolic effectors of the complex. It appears more likely, however, that these factors alter the kinase/phosphatase interaction with the enzyme. Among the potential effectors are the ATP/ADP, NAD/NADH, and acetyl-CoA/CoA ratios (Fig. 8.7). In general, substrates activate the complex and products cause its inhibition.

The acetyl-CoA generated by pyruvate dehydrogenase, by β oxidation of fatty acids, or by breakdown of certain amino acids then combines with oxaloacetate to form citrate. This reaction is catalyzed by *citrate synthase,* usually said to be the rate-limiting enzyme of the TCA cycle, and greatly favors citrate formation. There are several controls on the activity of this enzyme. The first is substrate availability and the second is succinyl-CoA, which is a competitive inhibitor of acetyl-CoA. The enzyme can also be inhibited by ATP and NADH *in vitro* but this may not be of physiological importance.

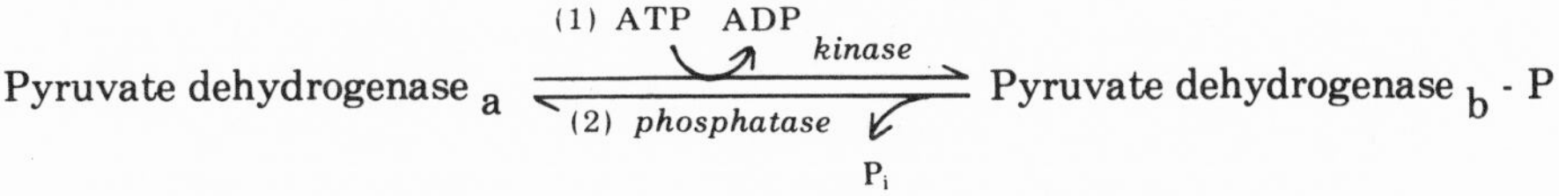

$$\text{Pyruvate dehydrogenase}_a \xrightarrow[\underset{P_i}{(2)\ \textit{phosphatase}}]{\overset{(1)\ \text{ATP}\ \ \text{ADP}}{\textit{kinase}}} \text{Pyruvate dehydrogenase}_b\text{-P}$$

Promotor	Inhibitor
(1) ATP	(1) dichloroacetate
low Mg^{2+}	ADP
	PP
(2) Ca^{2+}	pyruvate
high Mg^{2+}	Ca^{2+}
	(2) fluoride
	EGTA

FIG. 8.7.   Effectors of pyruvate dehydrogenase activity.

The citrate formed can be interconverted reversibly to isocitrate by *aconitase*. This essentially is a two part reaction composed of a dehydration to *cis*-aconitate and a rehydration to isocitrate. Aconitate is an enzyme bound intermediate and only a small amount (5%) becomes free in solution. Although citrate appears symmetrical, the reaction is stereospecific such that the water is added back to the portion of the molecule not derived from acetyl-CoA (Fig. 8.8).

The reaction is pulled toward isocitrate by the removal of isocitrate which in the next reaction is oxidized to α-ketoglutarate by *isocitric dehydrogenase*:

$$\text{isocitrate} + NAD^+ \rightarrow \alpha\text{-ketoglutarate} + NADH + H^+ + CO_2$$

There are two isozymes of isocitric dehydrogenase: one requires NAD and the other NADP. The NAD form is strictly mitochondrial and appears to be the enzyme involved in the TCA cycle. The NADP form, on the other hand is both mitochondrial and cytoplasmic. The NAD form has a requirement for ADP as a specific activator and also Mg^{2+}. ADP lowers the K_m of the enzyme for isocitrate. ATP and NADH are potent inhibitors of this enzyme. The isocitrate dehydrogenase reaction seems to be the secondary control point in the TCA cycle.

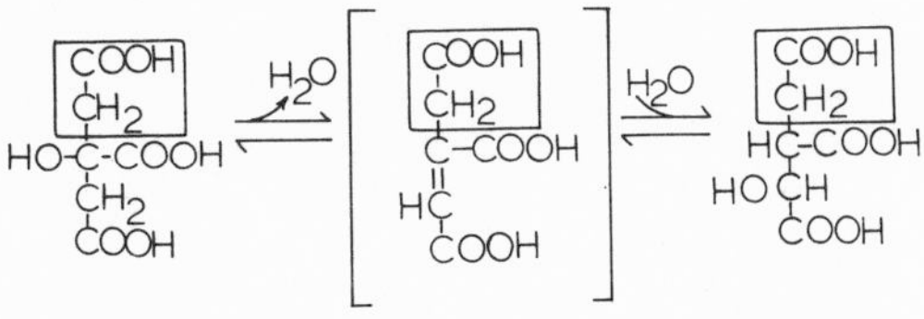

FIG. 8.8.   Aconitase reaction. The carbons in the boxes are derived from acetyl-CoA.

Citrate   Cis-aconitate   Isocitrate

The next step in the cycle is another oxidation. α-Ketoglutarate is oxidized to succinyl-CoA by *α-ketoglutarate dehydrogenase:*

$$\alpha\text{-ketoglutarate} + NAD^+ + CoA \rightarrow \text{succinyl-CoA} + CO_2 + NADH + H^+$$

This enzyme is very similar to the pyruvate dehydrogenase complex in that CoA, lipoic acid, FAD, NAD^+, and thiamine pyrophosphate are all required and the reaction mechanism is the same. Like pyruvate dehydrogenase, α-ketoglutarate dehydrogenase is quite a large complex. The NADP linked enzyme in *E. coli* has been shown to undergo phosphorylation. This may also prove to be the same case with the NAD-linked enzyme in mammals which would provide the final similarity with pyruvate dehydrogenase.

Once succinyl-CoA is formed, the energy in the thioester is conserved by what is known as a *substrate level phosphorylation.* In this reaction succinyl-CoA is hydrolyzed but the energy of the hydrolysis is conserved by converting GDP to GTP. The reaction, catalyzed by *succinyl-CoA synthetase,* is

$$\text{succinyl-CoA} + P_i + GDP \rightarrow GTP + CoASH + \text{succinate}$$

The resulting succinate contains the acetyl-CoA originally entering the TCA cycle, but since succinate is completely symmetrical, the location of the acetyl-CoA in succinate is randomized at this point.

Another oxidation comprises the next step in which succinate is oxidized to fumarate by *succinate dehydrogenase.* This reaction requires FAD rather than NAD as the electron acceptor, however.

$$\text{succinate} + FAD \rightarrow \text{fumarate} + FADH_2$$

The enzyme is tightly bound to the mitochondrial membrane and contains eight atoms each of iron and sulfur atoms which are acid labile. Although succinate dehydrogenase is not the rate-limiting enzyme in the TCA cycle, it is activated by succinate, phosphate, ATP, and reduced coenzyme Q and inhibited by low concentrations of oxaloacetate.

Next, *fumarase* catalyzes the reversible hydration of fumarate to L-malate:

$$\text{fumarate} + H_2O \rightarrow \text{L-malate}$$

Addition of water is always stereospecifically correct so that only L-malate is formed. The reaction is freely reversible.

The last reaction in the cycle is also an oxidation reduction step. The reaction involves malate which is oxidized by *malate dehydrogenase* which converts

$$\text{malate} + NAD^+ \rightarrow \text{oxaloacetate} + NADH + H^+$$

In addition to the mitochondrial form of malate dehydrogenase, which is associated with the TCA cycle in the mitochondria, there is also a cytoplasmic form of this enzyme. Although the equilibrium lies well toward malate, the reaction in the mitochondria proceeds toward oxaloacetate because of the rapid removal of oxaloacetate to combine with acetyl-CoA to form citrate.

Thus, in the complete TCA cycle, two carbons enter the cycle and two carbons become fully oxidized to CO_2. For any given turn of the cycle, it is, of course, not the same two carbons entering that are oxidized.

D. OXIDATIVE PHOSPHORYLATION

Although the TCA cycle serves to oxidize the carbons from carbohydrates, the reducing equivalents generated must be reoxidized with the energy of the oxidation being captured for use by the animal. This is accomplished by the electron transport chain which is a series of proteins in an array mostly tightly bound to the mitochondrial membrane. In the course of the reoxidation of NADH, ATP is generated at several steps along the way. The sequence is shown in Fig. 8.9. For substrates which produce NADH + H$^+$ upon being oxidized, the entry point of the electrons is at *NADH dehydrogenase,* a complex containing a flavoprotein and at least four iron–sulfur proteins. The next step

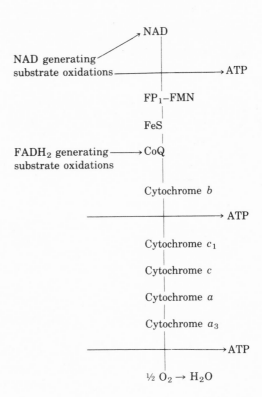

FIG. 8.9. Oxidative phosphorylation sequence.

involves transfer of electrons to coenzyme Q (ubiquinone). Substrates whose oxidations result in reduction of FAD → $FADH_2$ have electrons entering at the coenzyme Q step. From there, electrons traverse through the cytochromes b, c_1, c, a, and a_3. Cytrochromes b, c, and an iron–sulfur protein form the complex *ubiquinol dehydrogenase*. *Cytochrome oxidase* is comprised of cytochromes c, a, and a_3 and transfers electrons to oxygen to form water. ATP is generated by phosphorylating ADP at various steps along the way and is therefore "coupled" to oxidation. At a maximum, three ATP's are generated for each pair of electrons traversing the chains. The sites where ATP is generated are at the NADH dehydogenase step, the cytochrome b → c_1 step, and the cytochrome a → a_3 step. The exact coupling mechanism remains unknown. Phosphorylation can be uncoupled from oxidation by compounds such as dinitrophenol and dicumarol. When uncoupled, oxidation continues at a faster rate. Other compounds (e.g., rotenone) block electron transport, preventing oxidation and phosphorylation from occurring.

There are three current theories about the coupling between oxidation and phosphorylation. The earliest hypothesis was the chemical coupling model, which postulates the existence of a high energy intermediate used to convert ADP to ATP. Such an intermediate has not yet been discovered. Conformational coupling, another hypothesis, suggests that energy from electron transport is contained in a conformational change of some protein in the sequence. There is some evidence favoring this hypothesis, but it may be coincidental and is by no means conclusive. The third hypothesis is the chemiosmotic coupling theory for which Mitchell received a Nobel Prize. In this theory, a high energy state is believed to be generated as the result of pumping H^+ ions to form a gradient. Such a mechanism depends on the integrity of the mitochondrial membrane and impermeability of the membrane to hydrogen ion diffusion. Both of these conditions are met. Further, uncoupling agents increase membrane permeability, which is consistent with destruction of the proton gradient across the membrane. Additional research is needed to confirm the actual mechanism for coupling oxidation and phosphorylation.

E. AMINO ACID SYNTHESIS

Compounds entering the TCA cycle may escape the cycle before being completely oxidized to CO_2 and H_2O. For example, α-ketoglutarate may be transaminated to glutamate, and oxaloacetate may undergo the same fate to form aspartate. Alanine can be formed reversibly from pyruvate and serine; glycine, asparagine, and glutamine can also be made from glucose.

F. LIPID SYNTHESIS

Fatty acids and cholesterol are formed when blood glucose and insulin levels are high. In order for lipid synthesis to occur, there must first be a source of cytoplasmic acetyl-CoA. In nonruminants at least, this is accomplished by channeling some of the mitochondrial citrate into the cytoplasm via a hormone-sensitive carrier. The carrier is active when insulin levels are high. Citrate entering the cytoplasm is cleaved to oxaloacetate and acetyl-CoA by *ATP citrate lyase*. This is a rather involved reaction and requires ATP:

$$CoASH + citrate + ATP\text{-}Mg \rightarrow acetyl\text{-}CoA + ADP + P_i + oxaloacetate$$

The reaction is essentially irreversible *in vivo*. ATP citrate lyase, formerly called *citrate cleavage enzyme,* is active when insulin levels are high, such as with high carbohydrate diets and has low activity during fasting or diabetes. Unlike many other regulated enzymes, ATP-citrate lyase has few apparent metabolic effectors, and it has been difficult to rationalize its rapid regulation. Recently, however, it has become apparent that this enzyme belongs to the growing family of enzymes regulated by phosphorylation and dephosphorylation. There seems to be a further regulatory compensation in this system. If CoASH levels are high then the effect of phosphorylation on activity is overridden, whereas at low CoASH levels phosphorylation reduces the activity of the enzyme (Roehrig *et al.* 1982). There may be several sites of phosphorylation. The enzyme can be phosphorylated by cyclic AMP dependent and independent kinases.

The next enzyme in the sequence, *acetyl CoA carboxylase,* a biotin containing enzyme is generally believed to be the rate-limiting enzyme for fatty acid synthesis. It catalyzes the reaction

$$acetyl\text{-}CoA + HCOO^- + ATP\text{-}Mg \rightarrow malonyl\text{-}CoA + ADP + P_i$$

It has been well established that this enzyme is regulated by covalent modification. The enzyme is inactivated by phosphorylation and activated by dephosphorylation. Adding phosphate to the enzyme can be accomplished by both cyclic AMP dependent and independent kinases.

Citrate is a *potential* link regulating the relative activities of the pathway for fatty acid synthesis and glycolysis. High levels of citrate inhibit glycolysis at the phosphofructokinase step and accelerate the activity of acetyl-CoA carboxylase. This counterregulation would prevent the build up of intermediates if there was no place for them to go. It is doubtful, however, that control by citrate would be a "first-line" control device under normal physiological conditions because citrate levels are usually much lower than what is required for the effect.

The malonly-CoA generated by acetyl-CoA carboxylase is used by *fatty acid synthetase* to make fatty acids. The fatty acid that is preferentially produced in a particular tissue is dependent on the particular fatty acid synthetase in that tissue and on the ratio of acetyl-CoA to malonyl-CoA. High levels of malonyl-CoA favor the synthesis of longer chains. The overall reaction for the production of palmitate is

acetyl-CoA + 7 malonyl-S-CoA + 14 NADPH + 14 H$^+$ → palmitate + 7 CO$_2$ + 14 NADP$^+$ + 8 CoASH

Fatty acid synthetase is actually a large complex composed of six enzymes catalyzing a six-step sequence repetitively. In addition, acyl carrier protein (ACP) acts as the seventh protein portion and is a carrier for the growing fatty acid chain. The steps in sequence, with enzyme activities shown underneath in italics, are

1. acetyl CoA + ACP-SH ---→ acetyl-S-ACP + CoASH
   ACP acyltransferase
2. acetyl-S-ACP + synthetase-cysteine-SH → ACP-SH + acetyl-S-synthetase
   β-ketoacyl-ACP synthetase

These two reactions complete the "priming" part of the synthetase reaction.

3. malonyl-CoA + ACP-SH → malonyl-S-ACP + CoASH
   ACP malonyltransferase
4. acetyl-S-synthetase + malonyl-S-ACP → acetoacetyl-S-ACP + CO$_2$ + synthetase-SH
   β-ketoacyl ACP synthetase
5. acetoacetyl-S-ACP + NADPH + H$^+$ → β-hydroxybutyryl-S-ACP + NADP$^+$
   ketoacyl-ACP reductase
6. β-hydroxybutyryl-S-ACP → CH$_3$ CH=CH-C $\overset{O}{\sim}$ S-ACP + H$_2$O
   enoyl-ACP hydratase   (crotonyl-S-ACP)
7. crotonyl-S-ACP + NADPH + H$^+$ → butyryl-S-ACP + NADP$^+$
   enoyl-ACP hydratase

The cycle begins again when the butyryl group on the ACP is transfered to the cysteine of the synthetase and another malonyl-CoA is loaded onto the ACP portion of fatty acid synthetase. The newly formed fatty acids may then be esterified with glycerol to form triglycerides.

The NADPH necessary for fatty acid synthetase can come from the *hexose monophosphate shunt* (discussed later in this chapter), from *NADP linked isocitric dehydrogenase,* or from cytoplasmic *malic enzyme.* The oxaloacetate generated from the cleavage of citrate is converted to malate by cytoplasmic malate dehydrogenase. The malate thus generated is oxidatively decarboxylated to pyruvate and CO$_2$ with the reduction of NADP$^+$ to NADPH + H$^+$. Thus, oxaloacetate is not only channeled back to pyruvate but the reducing equivalents necessary for fat synthesis are produced at the same time.

Instead of being converted into fatty acids, acetyl-CoA derived from glucose can be channeled instead into cholesterol. The first step in this process is the formation of acetoacetate and then β-hydroxy-β-methylglutaryl-CoA (HMG-CoA) catalyzed by *HMG-CoA synthetase:*

acetyl-CoA + acetoacetyl-CoA ---→ β-hydroxy-β-methylglutaryl-CoA + CoA

The next step is the rate-limiting step for cholesterol synthesis. It is catalyzed by *HMG-CoA reductase,* a two-step reduction that is irreversible. The overall reaction catalyzed by reductase is

HMG-CoA + 2 NADPH + 2 H$^+$ ---→ mevalonate + 2 NADP$^+$ + CoA

HMG-CoA reductase activity shows a strong circadian rhythm with peak activity in the fed portion of the cycle (in rats this is around midnight but in nonnocturnal animals it would be in the daytime). Enzyme activity is highest when insulin levels are high and is lowest during periods of fasting or diabetes. HMG-CoA reductase is regulated by covalent modification (Fig. 8.10). Phosphorylation of the enzyme, which results inactivation, is controlled by reductase kinase, which itself can be reversibly phosphorylated and dephosphorylated. The reductase kinase is active when it is phosphorylated. The subsequent reactions of cholesterol synthesis are shown in Fig. 8.11. In the latter steps for cholesterol synthesis methyl groups are removed from lanosterol by successive oxidations. The preferred route from lanosterol to cholesterol is through 7-dehydrocholesterol although it is also possible to arrive at cholesterol via desmosterol.

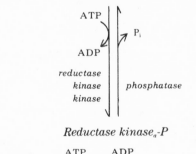

FIG. 8.10. Regulation of HMG-CoA reductase by covalent modification. Adapted from Ingebritsen and Gibson (1980).

G. HEXOSE MONOPHOSPHATE SHUNT

Instead of going through glycolysis and the TCA cycle to be completely oxidized or being shunted off to amino acid or lipid synthesis, some glucose may be shunted out of the glycolytic sequence very early at the glucose 6-phosphate step. At this point, glucose 6-phosphate can be mutated to glucose 1-phosphate or it can enter the *hexose monophosphate shunt* by being oxidized to 6-phosphogluconate. Only a small

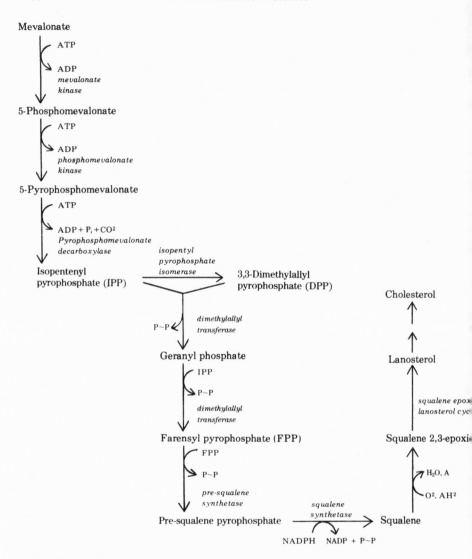

FIG. 8.11.   The reactions beyond HMG-CoA reductase leading to the production of cholesterol.

proportion of the glucose entering a tissue ultimately passes through the hexose monophosphate shunt (variously called the pentose shunt, phosphogluconate pathway, or pentose pathway), but this pathway is important for several reasons. First, it provides NADPH, which is necessary for lipid synthesis. Consequently, this pathway is most active in tissues where lipogenesis is high, i.e., liver, adipose tissue, mammary gland, and developing brain. Further, this pathway pro-

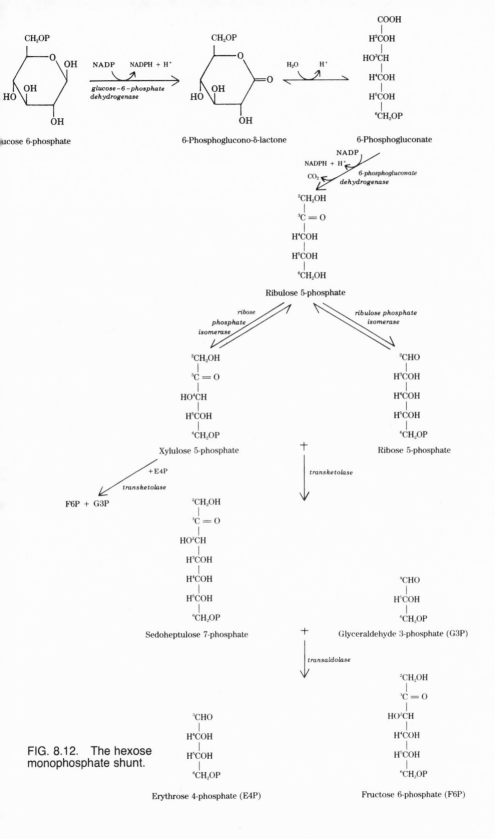

FIG. 8.12. The hexose monophosphate shunt.

duces ribose 5-phosphate necessary for the production of the various classes of RNA. The pathway is shown in Fig. 8.12. For each glucose entering only the C-1 is lost. Therefore, in order to get a stoichiometric balance for considering the equivalent of complete oxidation of glucose, i.e, the production of 6 CO_2, six turns of the cycle are needed. The balanced equation is as follows:

glucose 6-phosphate + 12 NADP$^+$ + 7 H_2O ---→ 6 CO_2 + 12 NADPH + 12 H$^+$ + P$_i$

If products are not channeled off for other uses (RNA, pentose formation, etc.) they will reenter the glycolytic pathway in the form of fructose 6-phosphate and glyceraldehyde 3-phosphate where they can continue being degraded.

All of the reactions of this pathway take place in the cytoplasm. The activity of the first enzyme in the shunt, glucose-6-phosphate dehydrogenase, is greatly stimulated by insulin and high carbohydrate diets and drops during fasting, diabetes, or when high fat diets are fed. Like the enzymes involved in lipogenesis, fasting followed by refeeding stimulates the activity well above control levels. This phenomenon is known as the *refeeding overshoot*. The other enzyme that is "coupled" to lipogenesis by virtue of its production of NADPH is *6-phosphogluconate dehydrogenase*.

The other most interesting reactions in the shunt are catalyzed by *transketolase* and *transaldolase*. Transketolase requires thiamine pyrophosphate. Two carbons are transferred from xylulose 5-phosphate (or any D-threo configured ketose) onto thiamine pyrophosphate, forming an active glycoaldehyde. This fragment is then transferred to a D-aldose. In the pathway either ribose 5-phosphate or erythrose 4-phosphate is an acceptor. As a result, if one were to specifically label the carbons of glucose, two types of fructose 6-phosphate would be found: one would be labeled 2-3-2-4-5-6 and the other would be 2-3-3-4-5-6.

Transaldolase is the other "interesting" enzyme in this pathway. It is similar to the aldolase in glycolysis and proceeds by the same mechanism (formation of a Schiff's base by interaction of the carbonyl of the substrate and an ε-amino group of a lysine on the enzyme). Unlike the glycolytic aldolase, however, it cannot form dihydroxyacetone.

H. GLYCOGEN SYNTHESIS AND DEGRADATION

Instead of entering the hexose monophosphate shunt, glucose 6-phosphate can be converted to glucose 1-phosphate by *phosphoglucomutase*. Next, the glucose 1-phosphate reacts with UTP to form UDP-glucose + P~P, a reaction catalyzed by *glucose-1-phosphate uridylyltransferase*. This reactive intermediate can go in several different directions. One route leads to the synthesis of glycogen.

Both the synthesis and degradation of glycogen will be considered together here because glycogen is not a static compound but is con-stantly being formed and broken down in response to the metabolic needs of an animal. Two tissues, liver and muscle, are especially important in glycogen metabolism. The liver, of course, is a major storage site of glycogen. After a fasting-refeeding cycle, the level of glycogen overshoots the control concentrations severalfold to the ex-tent that as much as 12% of the wet weight of liver is glycogen. The glycogen in liver serves as an important reserve of glucose which can be readily converted to blood glucose. Glycogen in muscle (up to 2% wet weight of muscle) serves a different purpose. Muscle is incapable of contributing glucose to the blood. Instead, muscle glycogen is broken down to provide energy for work under anaerobic conditions. The level of glycogen in muscle is little affected by fasting; depletion of this reserve is dependent on the amount and conditions of contraction of the muscle. One diet popular with some athletes in recent years is called "carbohydrate loading." This regimen seeks to build up large reserves of glycogen in the muscle, ostensibly to improve muscle performance.

Adipose tissue has nearly as much glycogen as muscle when one corrects for the weight of the lipid in the tissue. Since adipose also does not contribute glucose to blood, it may be supposed that in this case the glycogen serves as a source of glucose to be converted to α-glycerophosphate, which serves to reesterify fatty acids entering the adipose tissue from the blood.

High carbohydrate diets, insulin, and glucocorticoid administration promote glycogen synthesis whereas fasting, diabetes, and high fat diets result in glycogen breakdown. Study of the glycogen system has been the basis from which much of the knowledge about short-term regulation by covalent modification (phosphorylation/dephos-phorylation) has been derived.

The steps in the synthesis and degradation of glycogen are shown in Fig. 8.13. Much of what is known about the regulation of glycogen metabolism comes from studies on muscle. The system in liver is not entirely analagous. Where there are known differences, regulation of both systems will be discussed. The rate-limiting enzyme for synthesis is *glycogen synthetase* which occurs in an active (a) and an inactive (b) form. The interconversion between these two forms is caused by a phosphatase and a kinase(s). The molecular weight of glycogen syn-thetase has been reported to be from 140,000 to 500,000. It seems likely that the apparent disparity could be due to the presence or absence of regulatory proteins.

Glycogen synthetase activity is also dependent on the concentration of glucose 6-phosphate. In the older literature the inactive and active forms of the enzyme were labeled D and I, respectively. The D form is inactive unless considerable glucose-6 phosphate is present, but the I form is active in the absence of glucose 6-phosphate. Strictly speaking, the D/I nomenclature is not entirely analogous to the a/b designations. In any event, it is probably only the a(I) form which is active in liver.

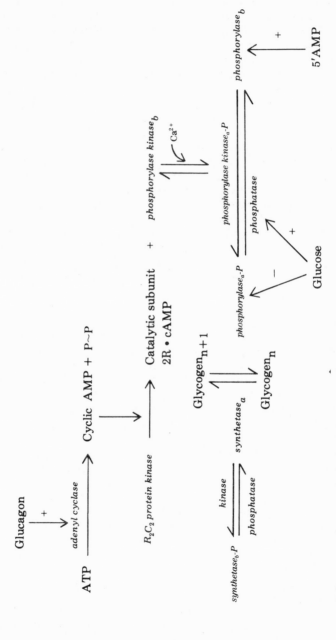

FIG. 8.13. Control of the synthesis and degradation of glycogen.

Regulation of the kinase side of the reaction may be more complex than first suspected. Initially, it was believed that cyclic AMP dependent protein kinase was responsible for the phosphorylation of glycogen synthetase. It was shown that sites designated 1a and 1b were phosphorylated as a result of the action of this kinase on glycogen synthetase. It has also been shown that phosphorylase kinase can phosphorylate a different site known as site 2. Recently, still a third kinase has been shown to be able to phosphorylate three additional sites (3a, 3b, and 3c) in the muscle system. There are still additional phosphorylation sites and additional kinases have been described (Cohen *et al*. 1982 and Picton *et al*. 1982). The physiological importance of this particular phosphorylation is not yet clear.

There are some other apparent regulatory features as well. The phosphatase side of the reaction also appears to be regulated. At this point, it seems likely that glycogen synthetase phosphatase and phosphorylase phosphatase are the same protein. Hence, when phosphatase is active, the synthesis side of the pathway is "on" and the degradation side is "off." Further, phosphorylase *a* is an inhibitor of phosphatase, so when the breakdown side is "on" the synthesis side will be "off." It has been postulated that the ability of glucocorticoids to stimulate glycogen synthesis is due to two factors: a stimulation of glycogen synthetase *a* and production of a factor which inhibits phosphorylase *a* inhibition of phosphate.

An additional form of regulation, the *in vivo* relevance of which has not yet been determined is the activation of synthetase by C-terminal proteolysis. A number of enzymes (including acetyl-CoA carboxylase) are activated by limited proteolysis. This may be proved in the future to be an important control mechanism. In this case the "clipping" occurs whether the starting material is phosphorylated or not. The net effect of this limited proteolysis is to make the enzyme more dependent on glucose 6-phosphate.

It appears that the phosphatase itself is also subject to regulation as well. There are two fractions of phosphatase; they have been designated I and II. Phosphatase I is regulated by two heat stable protein inhibitors, also designated I and II. Inhibitor I is only an inhibitor, however, after it has been phosphorylated by cyclic AMP dependent protein kinase. Inhibitor I inhibits phosphatase activity against all of its substrates. Insulin decreases the degree of phosphorylation of inhibitor I. Inhibitor II has a molecular weight between 25,000 and 30,000. It does not appear to be phosphorylated and it seems to affect the activity of phosphatase against all its substrates equally.

The phosphorylase side of the reaction is also regulated. There are some major differences between muscle and liver on this side of the pathway. Unlike muscle, which has a tetrameric phosphorylase, the liver enzyme is a dimer of approximately 185,000 MW. There is one pyridoxal phosphate per enzyme molecule. There is also one phosphorylatable serine/monomer. AMP has little effect on the liver enzyme. In muscle, however, AMP makes phosphorylase *b* nearly as active as phosphorylase *a*.

In the muscle system, glycogen breakdown cannot be initiated in the absence of calcium ions. At least one site for the calcium affect has been determined. Muscle phosphorylase kinase is a tetramer with a subunit structure $\alpha_4\beta_4\gamma_4\delta_4$ and a molecular weight of about one million. It has now been determined that the δ subunit of phosphorylase kinase is the calcium binding protein, calmodulin. The calmodulin is a permanent part of the phosphorylase kinase molecule, and when calcium binds to the δ subunit, the enzyme can become activated.

There are several phosphorylation sites on phosphorylase kinase. The β subunit is the regulatory subunit, the α subunit is catalytic, the γ subunit may be important in aligning other enzyme with muscle fibers, and, of course, the δ subunit is calmodulin. Both the α and β subunits become phosphorylated with at least two of the β subunits becoming phosphorylated before the α subunit phosphorylation commences.

There are apparently two phosphorylase kinase phosphatases. One is 170,000 MW and preferentially dephosphorylates α subunits. The other is 80,000 MW and dephosphorylates β subunits. Inactivation of phosphorylase itself is glucose dependent because glucose stimulates phosphatase and inhibits phosphorylase *a*.

I. SUMMARY

Glucose is an important metabolite in higher animals. It may be used immediately for energy production via the TCA cycle and oxidative phosphorylation or it may be stored as glycogen or fat for later use. Glucose is also the precursor for many important biological compounds, including other sugars and nonessential amino acids. The pathway by which glucose is metabolized is determined by the relative activities of the enzymes that use glucose as a substrate. These enzymes in turn are regulated by a variety of control mechanisms that respond to various physiological stimuli. Each pathway has one or more control points that determine the overall rate of the pathway. Certain key enzymes may be absent in some tissues, thereby determining to a greater degree what can happen to a given substrate. For example, except for liver and kidney, glucose-6-phosphatase is absent from tissues. This means that only liver and kidney can contribute glucose to the bloodstream and that all other tissues are glucose users if certain other conditions are met.

REVIEW QUESTIONS

1. Explain how the Cori cycle is involved in glucose homeostasis during anaerobic exercise.

2. What are the regulatory points in glycolysis?
3. Can cholesterol be synthesized entirely from glucose?
4. What is the rate-limiting step in the TCA cycle?

BIBLIOGRAPHY

Cohen, P. 1978. The role of cyclic AMP dependent protein kinase in the regulation of glycogen metabolism in mammalian skeletal muscle. Curr. Top. Cell. Regul. *14*, 118–196.
Cohen, P., Yellowlees, D., Aitken, A., Donnella-Deana, A., Hemmings, B., and Parker, R. 1982. Separation and characterization of glycogen synthetase kinase 3, glycogen synthetase kinase 4 and glycogen synthetase kinase 5 from rabbit skeletal muscle. Eur. J. Biochem. *124*, 21–35.
DePaoli-Roach, A., Roach, P., Pham, K., Kramer, G., and Hardesty, B. 1981. Phosphorylation of glycogen synthetase and of the B subunit of eukaryotic initiation factor two by a common protein kinase. J. Biol. Chem. *256*, 8871–8874.
Dunaway, G., and Segal, H. 1976. Purification and physiological role of a peptide stabilizing factor of rat liver phosphofructokinase. J. Biol. Chem. *251*, 2323–2329.
El-Maghrabi, M., Claus, T., Pilkis, J., Fox, E., and Pilkis, S. 1982. Regulation of rat liver fructose 2,6 bisphosphatase. J. Biol. Chem. *257*, 7603–7607.
Engstrom, L. 1978. The regulation of liver pyruvate kinase by phosphorylation-dephosphorylation. Curr. Top. Cell. Regul. *13*, 29–51.
Goldhammer, A., and Paradies, H. 1979. Phosphofructokinase: structure and function. Curr. Top. Cell. Regul. *15*, 109–141.
Hardie, G. 1981. Fat and phosphorylation. Trends Biochem. Sic. *6*, 75–77.
Hue, L., Blackmore, P., Shikama, H., Robinson-Steiner, A., and Exton, J. 1982. Regulation of rat liver fructose 2,6 bisphosphatase. J. Biol. Chem. *257*, 4308–4313.
Ingebritsen, T., and Gibson, D. 1980. Reversible phosphorylation of hydroxymethylglutaryl CoA reductase *In* Developments in Cell Regulation. P. Cohen, (Editor). Elsevier-North Holland Biomed. Press, Amsterdam, The Netherlands.
Ly, S., and Kim, K. H. 1981. Inactivation of hepatic acetyl CoA carboxylase by catecholamine and its agonists through the α-adrenergic receptors. J. Biol. Chem. *256*, 11585–11590.
Picton, C., Aitken, A., Bilham, T., and Cohen, P. 1982. Multi-site phosphorylation of glycogen synthetase from rabbit skeletal muscle. Eur. J. Biochem. *124*, 37–45.
Roehrig, K., Pope, T., and Uhal, B. 1982. Activity of ATP citrate lyase from insulin or glucagon treated hepatocytes. Fed. Proc., Fed. Am. Soc. Exp. Biol. *41*, 1461.
Storey, B., Lee, C., and Wikstrom, M. 1981. Is transmembrane electrochemical potential essential to mitochondrial energy coupling. Trends Biochem. Sci. *6*, 166–170.
Ureta, T. 1978. The role of isozymes in metabolism. Curr. Top. Cell. Regul. *13*, 233–258.
Van Schaftingen, E., Davies, D., and Hers, H.-G. 1982. Fructose 2,6 bisphosphatase from rat liver. Eur. J. Biochem. *124*, 143–149.
Wieland, O., Seiss, E., Weiss, L., Loffler, G., Patzelt, C., Portenhauser, R., Hartmann, U., and Schirmann, 1973. Structure function and regulation of the mammalian pyruvate dehydrogenase complex. *In* Rate Control in Biological Processes. Soc. Exp. Biol. *27*, 371–400.
Wilson, J. 1980. Brain hexokinase: the prototype ambiquitous enzyme. Curr. Top. Cell Regul. *16*, 1–44.

9

Synthesis of Glucose and Some Other Major Mono- and Disaccharides

A. GLUCONEOGENESIS

If glucose is not supplied by the diet, it can either be supplied from the breakdown of liver glycogen or generated by the liver or kidney from lactate, pyruvate, glycerol, or some of the amino acids. It is important to remember that breakdown of fatty acids by β oxidation results in the production of two carbon acetyl-CoA units, and that for every two carbons put into the TCA cycle, two carbons leave as CO_2. Therefore, there can be no net synthesis of glucose from fatty acids or from any compound that feeds into the acetyl-CoA pool such as certain amino acids.

The gluconeogenic pathway represents a reversal of the glycolytic pathway except that other enzymes are required to circumvent the irreversible steps in glycolysis. The overall pathway is shown in Fig. 9.1. During gluconeogenesis, all of the irreversible steps in glycolysis are blocked. Alternate enzymes are provided to bypass these blockages. It is similar to providing salmon with fish ladders so that they can get around dams to go upstream to spawn.

Glucokinase, phosphofructokinase, and pyruvate kinase are the enzymes that have decreased activity under conditions where gluconeogenesis is active, that is, during fasting, diabetes, or high fat feeding. Pyruvate carboxylase, PEP carboxykinase, fructose-1, 6-bisphosphatase, and glucose-6-phosphatase are the enzymes that are active under gluconeogenic conditions to circumvent the blockages.

Lactate and a number of amino acids feed in at the level of pyruvate. Since the pyruvate kinase reaction is irreversible, an alternate route must be used. Pyruvate dehydrogenase is also blocked so that option is closed. Mitochondrial acetyl-CoA under these conditions comes from the β oxidation of fatty acids and not via pyruvate dehydrogenase. Instead, pyruvate is carboxylated by *pyruvate carboxylase* to form oxaloacetate in the mitochondria. This reaction is

$$\text{pyruvate} + \text{ATP} + H_2O + HCO_3 \rightarrow \text{oxaloacetate} + P_i + \text{ADP}$$

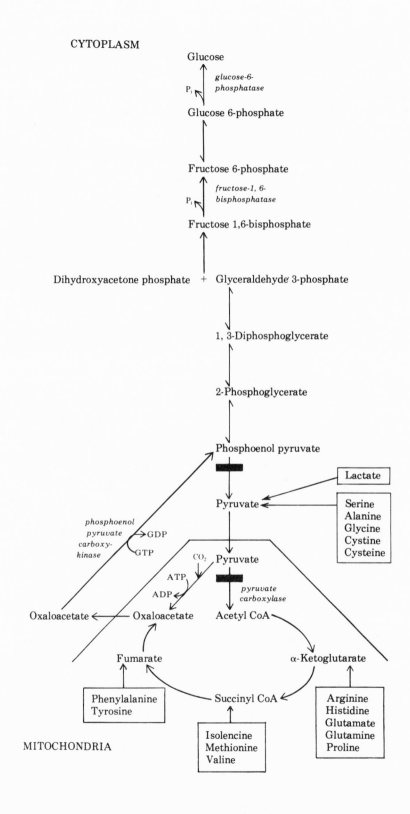

Pyruvate carboxylase is a biotin containing enzyme with the biotin attached to a specific lysine residue. The enzyme also requires K^+ and either or both Mg^{2+} and Mn^{2+}. In addition, pyruvate carboxylase is essentially inactive in the absence of acetyl-CoA. This helps to insure that gluconeogenesis will be active only when β oxidation is rapidly occurring, thus building up the pool of acetyl-CoA. In addition, control by acetyl-CoA level safeguards the continued functioning of the TCA cycle because if acetyl-CoA builds up because there is insufficient oxaloacetate to form citrate, then pyruvate carboxylase will be activated by the acetyl-CoA to form more oxaloacetate, ultimately resulting in the formation of citrate. Calcium is a potent inhibitor of pyruvate carboxylase by virtue of competitive inhibition with Mg^{2+}. Glutamate, at high levels ($K^+ > 5$ mM), is also an inhibitor but the physiological importance of this inhibition is doubtful.

After generation of oxaloacetate, the next step in gluconeogenesis is carried out by *PEP carboxykinase*. This step is complicated somewhat because there is a species dependent difference in distribution of this enzyme begween the cytoplasm and mitochondria. In mice and rats, this enzyme is cytoplasmic, in avian species and rabbits it is mitochondrial, whereas in humans, guinea pigs, and ruminants it is evenly distributed between the two compartments. Since oxaloacetate cannot escape from the mitochondria, in those species lacking mitochondrial PEP carboxykinase, oxaloacetate must first be converted to malate, exported on the malate aspartate shuttle to the cytoplasm, then reconverted to oxaloacetate by malate dehydrogenase before it can be acted upon by PEP carboxykinase. In species where the enzyme is mitochondrial, PEP is exported on a carrier directly without further conversion.

PEP carboxykinase catalyzes the reaction

$$\text{oxaloacetate} + \text{GTP} \rightarrow \text{PEP} + CO_2$$

Although GTP is the preferred nucleotide, others such as ITP will also work. The reaction is theoretically reversible, but physiologically its very low affinity for CO_2 renders it essentially irreversible.

It has been shown that PEP carboxykinase activity is enhanced by transition metal ions, particularly Fe^{2+}, Mn^{2+}, Co^{2+}, or Cd^{2+} (Lardy and Merryfield 1981). *In vivo*, iron seems to be the preferred ion. The activation of the enzyme by iron appears to be mediated by a large molecular weight (9×10^4 MW) protein called ferroactivator. The concentration of ferroactivator is highest when gluconeogenesis is "turned on," that is, during fasting, diabetes, and feeding of high fat diets. Ferroactivator apparently affects only the cytoplasmic form of the enzyme, even in species where a substantial portion of the enzyme may be mitochondrial. It was proposed that reaction of hormones with the

FIG. 9.1. Gluconeogenesis.

cell's α receptors causes calcium release from the mitochondria followed by Fe^{2+} release, binding of Fe to ferroactivator, then transfer of ferroactivator to PEP carboxykinase. On the basis of PEP carboxykinase inhibitor studies, it has been suggested (Rognstad 1979) that, at least under some conditions, PEP carboxykinase is a rate-limiting step in gluconeogenesis. Further studies will need to be done, however, to definitively demonstrate that this is indeed correct.

The next series of steps are reversals of the glycolytic pathway between PEP and fructose 1,6-bisphosphate. Once fructose 1,6-bisphosphate is formed, however, it cannot be converted to fructose 6-phosphate by phosphofructokinase since this enzyme catalyzes a physiologically irreversible step. Instead fructose-1,6-bisphosphatase catalyzes this conversion, thus circumventing the blockage. Inorganic phosphate is released and no ATP is formed.

Next, the fructose 6-phosphate is isomerized to glucose 6-phosphate. To produce glucose, it is necessary to bypass the irreversible glucokinase step. This is accomplished with the multifunctional microsomal

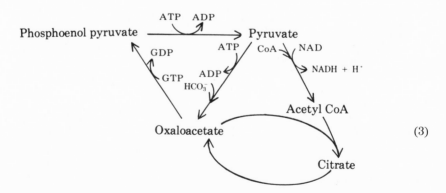

FIG. 9.2. Potential futile cycles between glycolytic and gluconeogenic enzymes.

enzyme, *glucose-6-phosphatase*. It is present only in liver and kidney. Its absence in muscle and adipose tissue accounts for why glycogen in these tissues is not a source of blood glucose. Like other membrane-bound enzymes, glucose-6-phosphatase is sensitive to its lipid environment.

The regulation of gluconeogenesis appears to occur by several mechanisms. One method of control is via cyclic AMP. Catecholamines functioning through cellular α receptors and other hormones, such as vasopressin and angiotensin II, apparently work via a cyclic AMP independent mechanism that may involve changes in calcium distribution. Insulin opposes the action of these agents.

The enzymes involved at potential control points in gluconeogenesis oppose control enzymes in glycolysis. If one enzyme is not "turned off" while the other is "turned on" then a futile cycle results which leads to the profiligate destruction of ATP. The potential futile cycles are shown in Fig. 9.2. It is likely that both sides of the reaction are controlled since this would provide for optimum metabolic regulation. There is some *in vitro* evidence that the pairs of enzymes involved in a potential cycle may be influenced by each other as well as by outside regulatory devices. For example, an interaction between phosphofructokinse and fructose-1,6-bisphosphatase has been observed in *in vitro* experiments.

B. GALACTOSE AND LACTOSE

Instead of going through glycolysis, glucose 6-phosphate can be converted to glucose 1-phosphate, which then reacts with UTP to form UDPglucose. Once UDPglucose is formed, galactose synthesis is a one step process. *UDPglucose-4'-epimerase* reversibly converts UDPglucose to UDPgalatose. This enzyme requires NAD^+, but $NADH + H^+$ is not produced as the result of the overall reaction. Instead an internal redox reaction occurs as shown in Fig. 9.3. The 4-keto derivative is formed then rereduced to the other UDPsugar.

For lactose formation it is necessary that UDPgalactose and glucose be available. Mammary gland has an enormous capacity to synthesize lactose. In human milk, the concentration of lactose is about 200 mM compared to a glucose concentration in the bloodstream of approx-

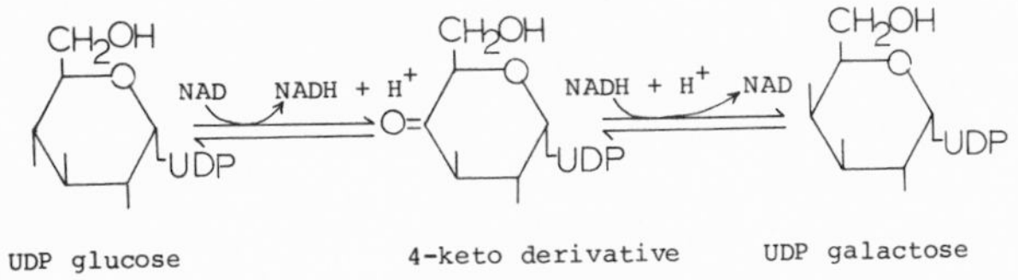

FIG. 9.3. Reaction mechanism for UDPglucose-4'epimerase.

imately 6 mM. The formation of lactose is catalyzed by *galactosyl-transferase*. A very unusual control system is operative in this case. Galactosyltransferase is present in most tissues, and yet lactose is produced only in the mammary gland. The usual substrates for the enzyme are UDPgalactose and N-acetylglucosamine. N-Acetyllactosamine, an important constituent of glycoproteins, is the normal product. In the mammary gland, however, a second protein is produced called α-lactalbumin. This protein combines with the transferase to change its substrate specificity by lowering the K_m for glucose so that glucose is used preferentially instead of N-acetylglucosamine.

Obviously, the mammary gland does not make lactose when milk is not being secreted. Prolactin, which is secreted during pregnancy by the anterior pituitary gland, is capable of stimulating the synthesis of both α-lactalbumin and galactosyl transferase. Lactose is not produced during pregnancy, however, because both the corpus luteum and the placenta secrete progesterone, which antagonizes the synthesis of α-lactalbumin. Once the fetus is delivered, the progesterone concentration falls allowing prolactin stimulation of the synthesis of these two proteins. Although lactose synthesis is important in the formation of most milk, milk from sea lions and certain other marine mammals contains essentially no carbohydrate.

C. AMINO SUGARS

Amino sugars play an important role in the function of a number of biological compounds. The formation of N-acetylglucosamine and UDP-N-acetylgalactosamine are shown in Fig. 9.4. Fructose 6-phosphate is the precursor and the nitrogen is donated from glutamine and the acetyl group is derived from acetyl-CoA. The UDP derivative is formed. UDP-N-Acetylglucosamine is an inhibitor of the first step in the pathway so, if for some reason it begins to accumulate, its synthesis ceases. The 4′-epimerase that converts UDP-N-acetylglucosamine to UDP-N-acetylgalactosamine is very much like the 4′-epimerase that converts UDPglucose to UDPgalactose in that it requires NAD^+ for an internal redox reaction.

UDP-N-acetylglucosamine also serves as the starting material for N-acetylneuraminic acid (sialic acid). The pathway is shown in Fig. 9.5. In order for sialic acid to be transferred to carbohydrate chains, it is necessary that it be transferred to CTP to form CMP N-acetylneuraminic acid.

D. UDPGLUCURONATE

UDPglucuronate is important for several reasons. It serves as the conjugating agent for the detoxification of a number of substances, and

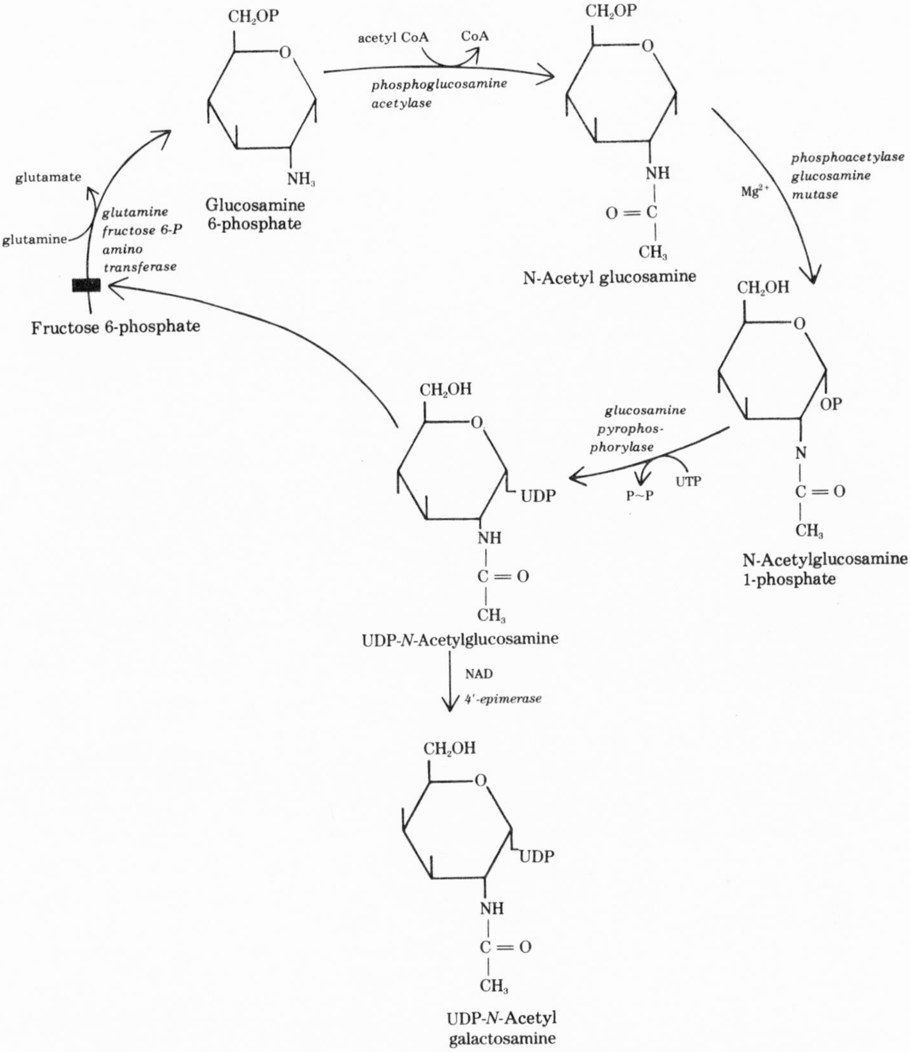

FIG. 9.4.   Formation of amino sugars.

is a precursor for ascorbic acid synthesis and for xylose formation. To synthesize UDPglucuronate a double oxidation catalyzed by *UDPglucose dehydrogenase* occurs. The reaction is

UDPglucose + 2 NAD$^+$ + H_2O → UDPglucuronate + 2 NADH + 2 H$^+$

The first oxidation converts the group on C-6 to an aldehyde and the second oxidation changes the aldehyde to a carboxyl carbon.

The detoxification of drugs using UDPglucuronate is principally a

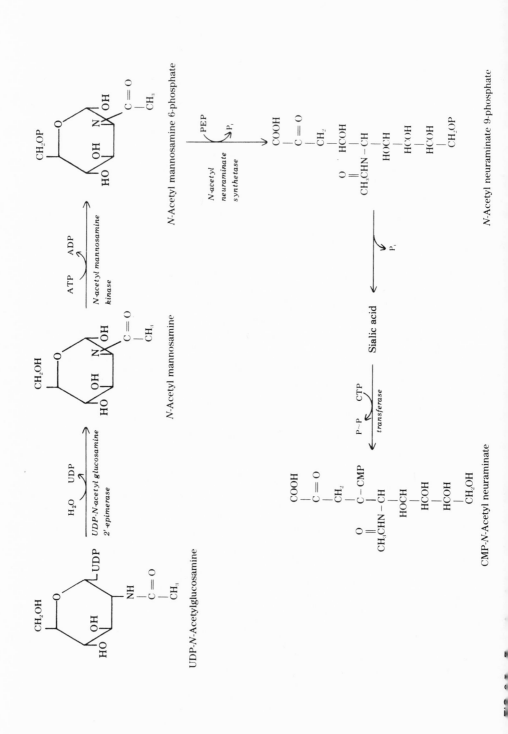

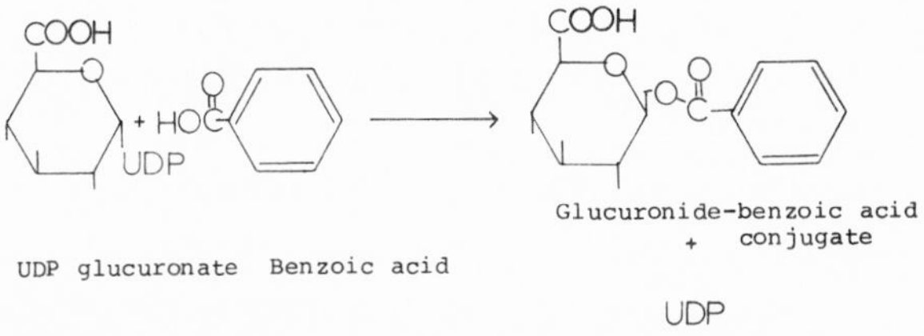

FIG. 9.6.   Glucuronide conjugation of benzoic acid.

liver reaction, catalyzed by glucuronyltransferase and includes conjugation of such compounds as phenols and amines. The general reaction is

$$\text{UDPglucuronate} + \text{ROH} \dashrightarrow \text{RO-glucuronide} + \text{UDP}$$

The UDP is always in the α configuration and the UDPglucuronate is
safe from attack by β-glucuronidase. The conjugates formed invariably
have a β configuration. The conjugation of benzoic acid by UDPglucuronate is shown in Fig. 9.6.

There are several glucuronyltransferases. The N-transferase is a
specific enzyme species. For example, bilirubin, a breakdown product
of hemoglobin, is detoxified by glucuronate conjugation. The Gunn rat
is genetically incapable of conjugating bilirubin, but it can perform
other glucuronate conjugations indicating the presence of multiple
species of the enzyme. This transferase reaction is microsomal and can
be stimulated by phenobarbital or DDT. Newborn babies often have
jaundice as the result of insufficient glucuronyltransferase activity to
conjugate the bilirubin. The problem can be partially overcome by
inducing the transferase with an agent like phenobarbital or UV light.

D-Glucuronic acid is also a presursor for ascorbic acid (vitamin C).
The pathway is given in Fig. 9.7. It occurs in plants and in the liver of
all higher animals except man, apes, guinea pigs, red vented bulbuls,
and Indian fruit bats. Even these species can complete the synthesis as
far as L-gulonolactone but lack L-gulonolactone oxidase, the final step
in making ascorbic acid.

UDPglucuronate is also a precursor of *UDPxylose*. Since xylose is
frequently found at the binding site of a polysaccharide to a peptide
core, this is an extremely important reaction. The reaction sequence is
shown in Fig. 9.8. If UDPxylose starts to build up, e.g., no protein core
is available, then the accumulated UDPxylose feeds back to inhibit the
first step in the reaction, UDPglucose dehydrogenase, thereby limiting
formation of UDPglucuronate. This would be expected to have several
consequences. Since UDPglucuronate is necessary for the conjugation
of a number of natural and foreign substances, this process would be
impaired. Further, in those animals capable of synthesizing ascorbic
acid, this pathway might also be compromised. In the usual *in vivo*

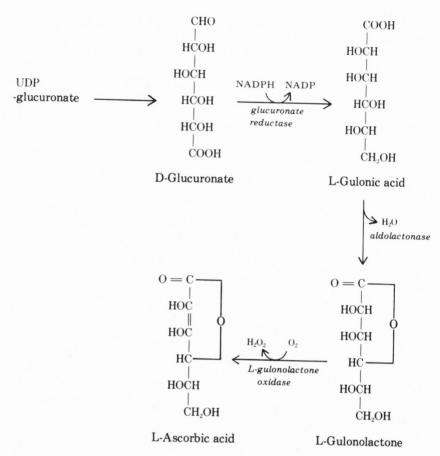

FIG. 9.7. Biosynthesis of ascorbic acid.

situation, however, such a regulatory device would seldom cause problems because an animal that is incapable of protein synthesis is in dire straits indeed and has such a host of other problems that one more does not signify. The inability to conjugate toxic materials or synthesize ascorbic acid, while certainly an additional insult, is likely to be the least of the animal's problems.

E. FRUCTOSE

Fructose formation is a process limited to a few specialized tissues such as the seminal vesicles, placenta, and lens of the eye. Since dietary fructose is efficiently trapped by the liver, little fructose is ever

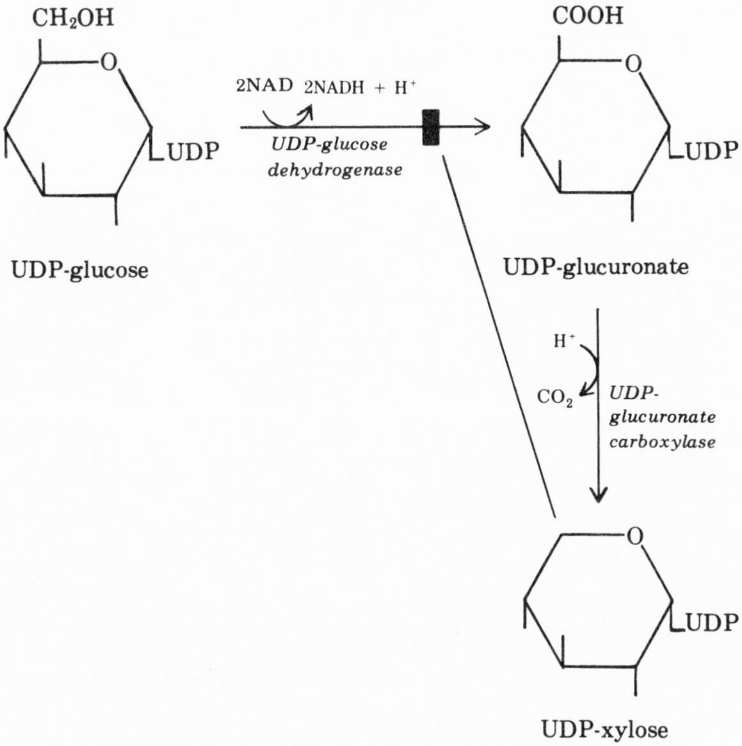

FIG. 9.8. Formation of UDPxylose.

found circulating in the blood. Most tissues except liver, kidney, and small intestine lack fructokinase and would have to rely on hexokinase to phosphorylate fructose. The utility of the hexokinase reaction for accomplishing this would depend on the levels of blood glucose. The specialized tissues, however (lens, placenta, and seminal vesicles), apparently have a need to provide a nutrient for endogenous use for which other tissues do not successfully compete. For example, the viability of sperm might be compromised under conditions of low blood glucose if glucose were its sole nutrient source. By using fructose synthesized in the seminal vesicles as a nutrient source, sperm would have a competitive edge over the surrounding tissues with regard to the nutrient supply.

The proposed pathway for the synthesis of fructose (Fig. 9.9) occurs via sorbitol. Free fructose is also found in fetal circulation and amniotic fluid of certain marine mammals and ungulates. Since there is no evidence that the livers of these animals can convert glucose to fructose, and since there is aldose reductase in the placenta, it is assumed

$$\text{D-Glucose} \xrightarrow[\substack{\text{NADPH}+\text{H}^+ \qquad \text{NADP}}]{\textit{Aldose reductase}} \text{D-Sorbitol} \xrightarrow[\substack{\text{NAD} \quad \text{NADH}+\text{H}^+}]{\textit{Sorbitol dehydrogenase}} \text{D-Fructose}$$

FIG. 9.9. Synthesis of fructose from glucose.

that the placenta is responsible for converting maternal blood glucose into fructose for use by the fetus to give the developing embryo an advantage in the battle for nutrient supplies.

F. SUCROSE SYNTHESIS

Animals cannot synthesize sucrose. Since sucrose is a major constituent in the food of humans and many other animals, however, its synthesis in plants will be briefly discussed. There are apparently two routes of formation (Fig. 9.10). One route involves making glucose 6-phosphate, mutating it to glucose 1-phosphate, then conjugating that to UDP to form UDPglucose. Simultaneously, fructose is phosphorylated to fructose 6-phosphate. The UDPglucose and fructose 6-phosphate react to form sucrose 6-phosphate. The phosphate is removed by a phosphatase to yield sucrose. The alternate pathway yields sucrose directly because UDPglucose is reacted with free fructose to form sucrose. Unlike the fructokinase in mammals, plant fructokinase gives fructose 6-phosphate rather than fructose 1-phosphate.

Although plants do not produce free glucose to any large extent, glucose is derived by photosynthesis from CO_2 via the Calvin cycle where CO_2 is fixed into 3-phosphoglycerate or via the Hatch–Slack pathway where CO_2 is fixed into four carbon dicarboxylic acids.

Route 1.
$$\text{ATP} + \text{Glucose} \xrightarrow{\text{hexokinase}} \text{Glucose-6-P} + \text{ADP}$$
$$\text{Glucose-6-P} \xrightarrow[\text{mutase}]{} \text{Glucose-1-P}$$

$$\text{UTP} + \text{Glucose-1-P} \xrightarrow[\text{G-1-P uridylyl-transferase}]{} \text{UDP-glucose} + \text{P}\sim\text{P}$$

$$\text{ATP} + \text{fructose} \xrightarrow[\text{fructokinase}]{} \text{Fructose-6-P} + \text{ADP}$$

$$\text{UDP-glucose} + \text{fructose-6-P} \xrightarrow[\text{sucrose phosphate synthetase}]{} \text{Sucrose-6-P}$$

$$\text{Sucrose-6-P} + \text{H}_2\text{O} \xrightarrow[\text{phosphatase}]{} \text{Sucrose} + \text{P}_i$$

Route 2.
$$\text{UDP-glucose} + \text{fructose} \xrightarrow[\text{sucrose synthetase}]{} \text{UDP} + \text{Sucrose}$$

FIG. 9.10. Sucrose synthesis.

G. SUMMARY

Gluconeogenesis is the method whereby glucose can be supplied by the liver or kidney to the bloodstream by the conversion of glycogen or lactate, pyruvate, glycerol, or certain amino acids into glucose. Gluconeogenesis operates by the reversal of glycolysis except at the irreversible rate-limiting steps where alternate enzymes are provided. These alternate enzymes are pyruvate carboxylase, PEP carboxykinase, fructose-1, 6-bisphosphatase and glucose-6-phosphatase. When gluconeogenesis is operative (fasting, diabetes, and high fat diets) then the rate-limiting steps in glycolysis (glucokinase, phosphofructokinase, and pyruvate kinase) are turned off. If both sides of the reaction occurred at the same time, futile cycling would result and ATP would be wasted. PEP carboxykinase is probably the overall rate-limiting enzyme.

Galactose is synthesized from glucose by an epimerization of UDPglucose by an internal oxidation and reduction. Lactose is produced by combining UDPgalactose with glucose in an enzyme reaction catalyzed by galactosyltransferase. Normally this enzyme catalyzes N-acetyllactosamine formation from UDPgalactose and N-acetylglucosamine. A second protein, α-lactalbumin combines with the transferase to change its specificity from N-acetylglucosamine to glucose thereby causing lactose to be produced.

Another very important synthetic product is UDPglucuronate produced by a double oxidation of UDPglucose. It has an extremely important role in the detoxification of a number of compounds by forming the glucuronide conjugate of the waste product. UDPglucuronate is also the precursor for vitamin C in most animals. It is also important in synthesis of glycoproteins because it is the precursor for vitamin C in most animals. It is also important in synthesis of glycoproteins because it is the precursor for UDPxylose, which is often the monosaccharide that attaches a polysaccharide chain to a protein core.

REVIEW QUESTIONS

1. What are the rate limiting enzyme(s) of gluconeogenesis?
2. What is ferroactivator?
3. What is the configuration of glucuronide conjugates and what functions do they serve?
4. By what mechanism is galactosyltransferase altered to produce lactose?

BIBLIOGRAPHY

Cherrington, A. 1981. Gluconeogenesis: its regulation by insulin and glucagon. *In* Diabetes Mellitus, Vol. III. M. Brownlee (Editor). Garland STPM Press, New York.
Claus, T., and Pilkis, S. 1981. Hormonal control of hepatic gluconeogenesis. *In* Bio-

chemical Actions of Hormones, Vol. VIII. G. Litwack (Editor). Academic Press, New York.

Exton, J. 1979. Hormonal control of gluconeogenesis. Adv. Exp. Med. Biol. *111*, 125–167.

Hanson, R., and Mehlman, M. 1976. Gluconeogenesis: its regulation in mammalian species. J. Wiley & Sons, New York.

Horecker, B., MacGregor, J., Singh, V., Melloni, E., and Pontremoli, S. 1981. Aldolase and fructose bisphosphatase: key enzymes in the control of gluconeogenesis and glycolysis. Curr. Top. Cell. Regul. *18*, 181–197.

Lardy, H., and Merryfield, M. 1981. Ferroactivator and the regulation of gluconeo-genesis. Curr. Top. Cell. Regul. *18*, 243–254.

Merryfield, M., Kramp, D., and Lardy, H. 1982. Purification and characterization of a rat liver ferroactivator with catalase activity. J. Biol. Chem. *257*, 4646–4654.

Rognstad, R. 1979. Rate-limiting steps in metabolic pathways. J. Biol. Chem. *254*, 1875–1978.

10

Metabolism of Complex Carbohydrates

A. INTRODUCTION TO POLYSACCHARIDE SYNTHESIS

Sugar nucleotides play a central role in polysaccharide synthesis. A number of monosaccharide units are transferred to growing carbohydrate chains with the aid of various sugar nucleotides. In Chapter 8, the synthesis of glycogen was described, in which uridine, in the form of uridine diphosphate, was the carrier. In the synthesis of other polysaccharides, however, the uridine may be replaced by adenosine, cytidine, guanosine, or thymidine.

The general reaction for polysaccharide synthesis occurs in two stages. The first is the action of a kinase on a monosaccharide to form a sugar phosphate, and the second is the interaction of the sugar phosphate with a nucleotide triphosphate to form pyrophosphate and the nucleotide diphosphate–sugar complex. The pyrophosphate is derived from the α and β phosphates of the nucleotide triphosphate. Once the sugar nucleotide is formed, it can be transferred to other sugars or sugar polymers.

It is interesting to note the similarities in the formation of glycogen and starch, cellulose, or chitin. Although different nucleotides are involved (Fig. 10.1), reaction sequences to form the ultimate products are similar to the synthetic reactions for glycogen. Amylopectin, the

A. Starch

$$\text{ATP} + \alpha\text{-Glucose-1-P} \quad \rightarrow \text{ADP-glucose} + P{\sim}P$$
$$\text{ADP-glucose} + \text{Glucose}_n \rightarrow \text{ADP} + \text{Glucose}_{n+1}$$

B. Cellulose

$$\beta\text{-Glucose-1-P} + \text{GTP} \quad \rightarrow \text{GDP glucose} + P{\sim}P$$
$$\text{GDP-glucose} + \text{glucose}_n \rightarrow \text{GDP} + \text{glucose}_{n+1}$$

C. Chitin

$$\text{UDP-}N\text{-acetyl glucosamine} + N\text{-acetyl glucosamine}_n \rightarrow$$
$$\text{UDP} + \beta(1{\rightarrow}4)N\text{-acetyl glucosamine}_{n+1}$$

FIG. 10.1. Syntheses of starch, cellulose, and chitin.

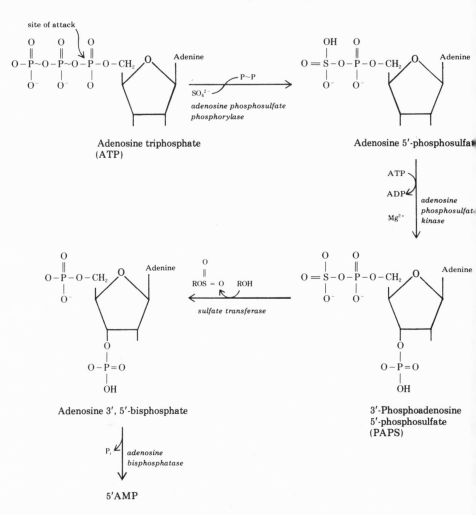

FIG. 10.2.   Sulfate transfer to carbohydrates.

branched form of starch, also requires the action of a branching enzyme to transfer sections of α (1→4) chains to α (1→6) positions.

B. SULFATION OF POLYSACCHARIDES

Many of the complex carbohydrates are sulfated. Sulfation appears
to occur in the same way regardless of the composition of the carbohydrate. Further, it seems that sulfate is usually added to the preformed
complex carbohydrate rather than by addition of sulfate to a monomer.

Most of the sulfate for this purpose comes ultimately from sulfate derived from the degradation of the sulfur amino acids, cysteine and methionine, but some will be obtained from the diet as inorganic sulfate. In order to be added to carbohydrates, the sulfate must first be activated to 3'-phosphoadenosine 5'-phosphosulfate (PAPS), a mixed anhydride which is a high energy compound. PAPS formation requires two steps (Fig. 10.2): generation of adenosine 5'-phosphosulfate and then phosphorylation of this compound to form PAPS catalyzed by a kinase. PAPS donates its sulfate to an acceptor in a reaction catalyzed by sulfate transferase, leaving adenosine 3',5'-bisphosphate, which should not be confused with adenosine 3',5'-monophosphate (cyclic AMP), which has only one phosphate group cyclized between the 3' and 5' hydroxyl groups. When the breakdown product of PAPS is further degraded by adenosine bisphosphatase, 5'-adenosine monophosphate and inorganic phosphate are formed. On the other hand, when cyclic AMP is degraded, the reaction is catalyzed by cyclic AMP phosphodiesterase and the product is only 5'-adenosine monophosphate.

C. METABOLISM OF MUCOPOLYSACCHARIDES

Mucopolysaccharides are increasingly referred to as glycosaminoglycans. The most abundant of this class is hyaluronic acid, which is abundant in cellular ground substance and in synovial fluid. There is some evidence that some patients with rheumatoid arthritis have higher levels of hyaluronic acid in the joint fluid than normal but that the hyaluronic acid is not completely polymerized. Perhaps, incorrectly polymerized hyaluronic acid impairs joint function. The higher levels could be the result either of impaired synthesis or increased degradation. There is an increased amount of *hyaluronidase* in the synovial fluid of rheumatoid arthritics which may give rise to an increased degradation. Hyaluronidase breaks down hyaluronic acid by randomly hydrolyzing the 1→4 linkages between acetylglucosamine and glucuronate and can also degrade chondroitin and dermatan sulfates. Treatment with hydrocortisone returns the degree of hyaluronic acid polymerization to normal.

Although some physiological reducing agents (cysteine, L-ascorbate, etc.) can also cause polymerization, the regulation of the synthesis and degradation of this mucopolysaccharide is still imperfectly understood. Two synthetic schemes have been proposed but neither has been proved (Fig. 10.3). The first scheme is a one step at a time approach and the second scheme is condensation of two unit fragments. Further experimentation is required to determine which if either of these modes of synthesis is operative *in vivo*.

Other important glycosaminoglycans include the chondroitins and heparin. Chondroitin sulfates A and C, chondroitin 4-, and chondroitin 6-sulfates, respectively, are very similar in structure and are found in

Scheme 1.
1. UDP glucuronate + N-acetylglucosamine-1-P →
   Glucuronate-N-acetylglucosamine-1-P + UDP
2. UDP-N-acetylglucosamine + glucuronate-N-acetylglucosamine-1-P →
   N-acetylglucosamine-glucuronate-N-acetylglucosamine-1-P + UDP
Scheme 2.
1. UDP-N-acetylglucosamine + UDP glucuronate →
   N-acetylglucosamine-glucuronate UDP + UDP
2. N-acetylglucosamine-glucuronate-UDP + N-acetylglucosamine-glucuronate-UDP →
   N-acetylglucosamine-glucuronate-N-acetylglucosamine-glucuronate -UDP + UDP

FIG. 10.3. Potential pathways for the synthesis of hyaluronic acid.

cartilage, bone, and tumors of connective tissue. Chondroitin sulfate C is also found in the umbilical cord and B and C together are found in mammalian heart valves. Unsulfated chondroitin is in the cornea. The synthesis of chondroitins occurs via nucleotide sugars as is common to the synthesis of complex carbohydrates. The chains can be synthesized entirely from glucose as would be predicted. It is generally agreed that the sulfation of chondroitin with PAPS as the sulfate donor occurs on the preformed chondroitin rather than on the monomeric units.

The sulfated chondroitins can also be physically linked with protein to form chondromucoprotein, which is found largely in the nasal passages. The linkage is via a serine residue. There is a neutral trisaccharide (galactose-galactose-xylose) interposed between the chondroitin and the protein. There must be considerable regulation involved in the synthesis and binding of chondroitins to protein because each tissue and species have quite different but self-consistent amounts of chondroitin sulfate and/or other mucopolysaccharides and also have consistent molecular weights.

Undoubtedly, much of the regulation must be hormonally controlled. Insulin and somatomedins both stimulate synthesis of cartiage glycoproteins [for a review see Stevens et al. (1981)]. There are increases in sulfate incorporation and in protein synthesis as well.

Chondroitin sulfate B, dermatin sulfate, is particularly associated with the skin and presumably is synthesized in a manner similar to chondroitin sulfates A and C. Since dermatin sulfate contains iduronic acid this must, of course, be synthesized first from UDPglucuronic acid (Fig. 10.4). Unlike the A and C forms, however, the B form is quite resistant to degradation by hyaluronidase. Lysosomal degradation of chondroitins by glycosidases is probably the most important route for their removal.

Heparin (named after hepatic tissue where it was first discovered) is an anticoagulant and an antilipemic agent usually bound to tissue protein. It has been used successfully in the treatment of heart disease. Heparin originates and/or is stored in mast cells, which are found mainly in connective tissue near capillaries and in vessel walls. Ordinarily, very little heparin is found free in circulation. In the mast

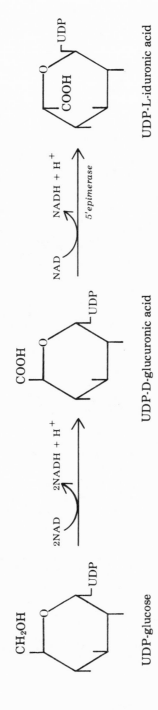

FIG. 10.4. Synthesis of L-iduronic acid.

cells, heparin is found associated with histamine. When heparin is associated with cellular protein, it is probably via a xylosyl-serine linkage. In anaphylactic shock, heparin and histamine are released into circulation from their locations in intracellular granules.

Once into circulation, heparin exerts its anticoagulant action by inhibiting the formation of thromboplastin and the action of thrombin. It also has fat clearing (antilipemic) activity. Normally, animals consuming a fatty meal will have turbid plasma because of the presence of chylomicrons and low density lipoproteins in the blood. Injection of heparin i.v. clears the plasma within a few minutes. This effect cannot be duplicated *in vitro* unless plasma from a previously heparin treated animal is used. Thus, a clearing factor (clearing factor lipase) is induced by heparin treatment. Actually the total fat content of the blood does not really change but the fatty acids become bound to albumin resulting in "clearing" of the plasma.

Although the complete synthesis scheme of heparin has not been elucidated, it is known to occur via nucleotide sugars with PAPS as the sulfate donor. The synhesis sequence outlined by Riesenfeld *et al.* (1982) is (1) polymer formation, (2) N-deacylation, (3) N-sulfation, (4) C-5 epimerization, and (5) O-sulfation. As in other cases, sulfate is not added until the carbohydrate chain is completely formed. The breakdown of heparin is equally uncertain. No endogenous heparinases have been found to date, but bacteria in the G.I. tract are capable of degrading heparin. Part of the uncertainty about the synthesis and degradation of heparin arises because of its extreme heterogeneity. There are at least 22 naturally occurring heparin chains, many of which do not possess anticoagulant activity. It has been suggested by Jaques (1979) that some chains may well have other, as yet unknown, functions.

D. METABOLISM OF GLYCOPROTEINS

The synthesis and degradation of glycoproteins are of extreme interest because of the broad range of functions of these compounds and the immense importance of these functions to the well-being of the organism. Cell recognition, host defense, hormones, and hormone receptors are just a few of the roles of glycoproteins.

Although there is great diversity in the protein component of glycoproteins, there is rather less in the carbohydrate portion. Only about nine out of more than 100 carbohydrates usually appear in the carbohydrate portion of glycoproteins. Also, the carbohydrate chains are not very long, usually less than 15 residues. The more common carbohydrate constituents in glycoproteins are acetylglucosamine, fucose, acetylgalactosamine, arabinose, xylose, galactose, mannose, and neuraminic acid. Unsubstituted glucose is rarely found in this class of compounds. Bunn and Higgins (1981) suggested that the stable ring structure of glucose makes it a good metabolic fuel and less likely to glycosylate proteins. On the other hand, those sugars that are found more often in open conformation are better substrates for glycosylation reactions but would be poorer fuels because of the competition for glycosylation reactions.

The synthesis and catabolism of glycoproteins have been presented in an excellent review by Schachter, Narasimhan, and Wilson (1978). There are several types of linkages between carbohydrates and proteins. One of the most common linkages between carbohydrate and protein, shared by many of the secreted glycoproteins, is the N-glycosidic linkage formed between asparagine and *N*-acetylglucosamine. The linkage type itself is an important control point that determines the type of carbohydrate chain that will ultimately be attached to the protein. Thus, there tends to be a set of common chains that subsequently attach to a particular glycosidic linkage. The asparagine-linked class of glycoproteins falls into three structural patterns: (1) one containing only mannose and *N*-acetylglucosamine, (2) heterosaccharides with more than two types of carbohydrate, and (3) a hybrid of (1) and (2). Most, however, share a common chain near the protein (Fig. 10.5). This particular class of carbohydrate linkage differs from the others in its formation in that the carbohydrate chains are assembled on a lipid carrier and, when completed, are transferred to the appropriate protein asparagine residue. The lipid carrier is a polyprenol compound, dolichol phosphate. Although dolichol does occur in the diet, endogenous synthesis probably provides most of the body pool of this compound (Keller *et al.* 1982). The synthesis of dolichol phosphate has been shown to occur on the outer mitochondrial membrane from mevalonate, and dolichol phosphate synthetase appears to be the rate-limiting enzyme. Dolichol phosphate may also be formed from free dolichol and CTP by the action of a kinase. The equilibrium between the two is also determined by dephosphorylation reactions. Recently, Carson and Lennarz (1981) suggested that the rate of dolichol synthesis itself is important in regulating the rate of protein glycosylation at least in embryonic sea urchins. When the rate of dolichol synthesis was inhibited by compactin (a competitive inhibitor of HMG-CoA reductase), protein glycosylation was also inhibited and the carbohydrate chains that were synthesized and attached to protein were altered compared to normal controls. A group of nucleoside antibiotics,

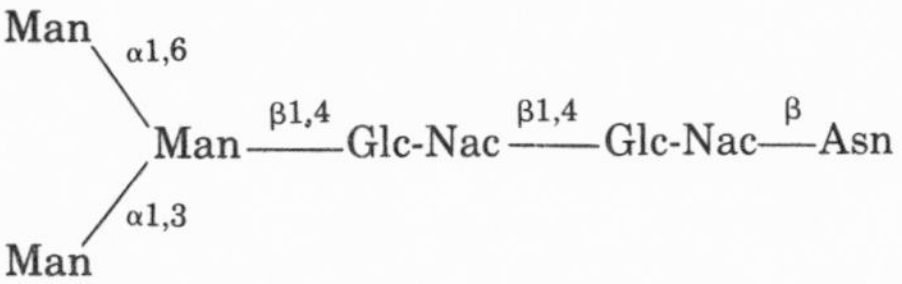

FIG. 10.5. The common chain of asparagine linked glycoproteins.

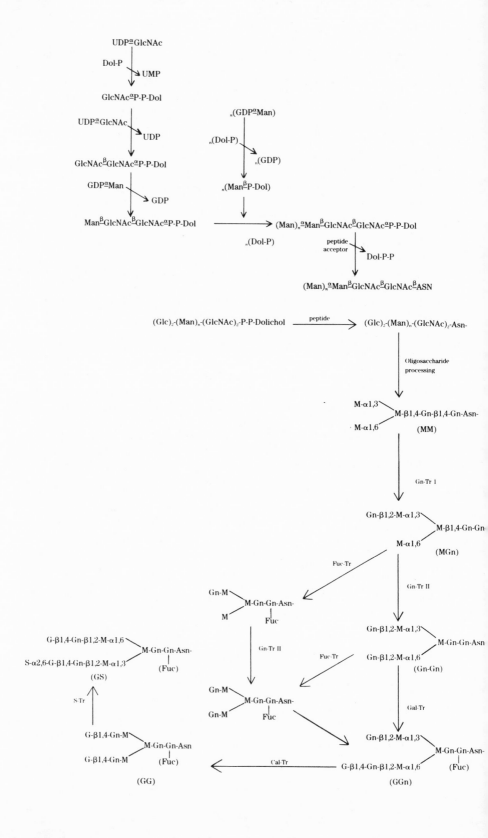

the tunicamycins (Elbein 1981), also impair glycoprotein synthesis. In eukaryotes, it is the first step that is blocked, i.e., the transfer of N-acetylglucosamine 1-phosphate from UDP-N-acetylglucosamine to dolichol phosphate. Tunicamycin, produced by *Streptomyces* does not appear to inhibit subsequent steps of chain elongation or addition of any other than the first N-acetylglucosamine to the protein. Use of these inhibitors has become a valuable tool in assessing the role(s) of carbohydrates in glycoprotein structure, function, and half-life.

Another common type of bond is a glycosidic linkage between N-acetylgalactosamine and serine or threonine. Other sugars that may be linked in this way are xylose, mannose, galactose, and fucose. Galactose may be bonded to hydroxylysine, hydroxyproline, or cysteine. This type of bond is common in collagen structures and certain membranes.

The amino acid sequences around the carbohydrate binding sites are known for quite a number of glycoproteins [for a listing see Waugh and Bahl (1981)]. For N-glycosidic linkages to asparagine there appears to be an invariant amino acid sequence [Asn-X-Thr(Ser)]. There does not, however, appear to be a common pattern for the serine and threonine glycosidic linkages. The synthesis of a polysaccharide linked to dolichol for transfer to an asparagine has been outlined (Fig. 10.6). Some further alterations of the carbohydrate chain can occur once it is attached to the protein. The core chain can undergo elongation or processing of the constituents of the chain.

There is still some conflict as to what point in time the carbohydrate chain is attached to a protein. Some researchers have found significant incorporation of carbohydrate into newly made protein strands while the nascent proteins are still attached to the ribosomes. Others do not agree, but all were studying different types of proteins. Since the transferase that removes oligosaccharide from the dolichol carrier and transfers it to protein is present in the highest concentration in rough endoplasmic reticulum, it must be assumed that the transfer process occurs close to the time when the protein chain is being formed.

Synthesis of serine (threonine) glycosidic linkages is substantially different from the asparagine case described above. In this instance no lipid carrier intermediate is formed. First, N-acetylgalactosamine is transferred from UDP-N-acetylgalactosamine to a protein acceptor. If the next carbohydrate added is sialic acid (from CMP sialic acid), further incorporation ceases (Fig. 10.7). If, however, a galactose is added, the carbohydrate chain can be further elongated.

The degradation of glycoproteins is also an important event. The sugars may be removed one at a time from the nonreducing end. There

FIG. 10.6.   Synthesis of a lipid linked carbohydrate chain for the transfer of carbohydrate to an asparagine of a protein chain.
Reprinted with permission from Schachter et al. (1978). Copyright 1978 American Chemical Society.

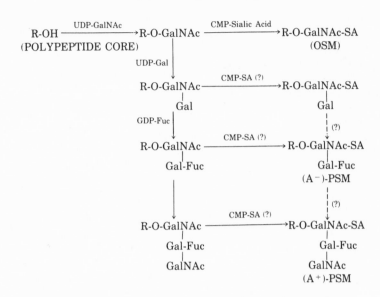

FIG. 10.7.   Synthesis of serine (threonine) type glycoproteins.
Reprinted with permission from Schachter et al. (1978). Copyright 1978 American Chemical Society.

are also endoglucosidases, which hydrolyze the carbohydrate in the interior portions of the chain. In some cases, loss of part or all of a carbohydrate chain may signal the demise of a glycoprotein. For example, a number of serum proteins have a terminal sialic acid. If this is removed, a galactose is exposed. Liver can then remove this protein from circulation and degrade it if the protein binds to a surface receptor that recognizes galactose. For example, ceruloplasmin normally has a half-life of 54 hr but removal of any two of 10 of its sialic acid residues reduces its half-life to minutes. The livers of birds and reptiles generally do not remove the protein at the stage when only sialic acid residues have been degraded. In these species, the galactose must also be removed exposing the third residue, *N*-acetylglucosamine, for which there are liver receptors.

The terminal ends of the carbohydrate chains on glycoproteins appear to be enormously important in normal cell function and cell recognition processes. The outside surfaces of cells are literally covered with carbohydrate. Lectins from one cell can bind to the carbohydrates on the surface of another cell forming bridges between them. Cells recognize other cells as "self" or "nonself" due in part to the nature of their carbohydrates. In fact, some cells have the capacity at certain stages in their cell cycles to mask themselves in such a way as to be invisible to host defenses. Some tumor cells can coat themselves with large quantities of sialic acid-containing glycoproteins making the tumor cells seem like normal cells. It may be that clinical use can be made of special tumor secreted glycoproteins. α-Fetoprotein, for example, is found in high concentrations in fetal serum but is virtually absent in normal adult serum. When an individual has malignant liver tumors, however, there is again a rise in α-fetoprotein. Identification of such markers in sera may prove to be valuable diagnostic markers for liver cancer screening and for prognosis after treatment.

In the next few years, the study of cell surface glycoproteins will undoubtedly yield a wealth of information about the way in which cells interact with each other and about methods to keep them from acting inappropriately. The role of glycoproteins in cellular receptors for various hormones will also be an increasingly important area for investigation. Use of lectins, carbohydrate binding proteins, will make this area of research rather more easy to deal with than it has been in the past. For example, concanavalin A from jack beans has already been useful in studying insulin interaction with cells. When concanavalin A binds to a cell, the cell behaves just as if insulin were bound to it instead. Concanavalin A is known to bind to carbohydrates with a D-arabino configuration. Studies such as these are useful in determining the structural features of hormone receptors.

E. SUMMARY

A common feature in the synthesis of most carbohydrate chains is first the formation of a sugar phosphate and next the reaction of the sugar phosphate with a nucleotide triphosphate to form a nucleotide diphosphate–sugar complex. Chains are progressively built up this way and branches are made by removing sections of preformed chain to appropriate branch points.

Synthesis of mucopolysaccharides has not been completely elucidated but several facets seem clear. The sulfation of these compounds, for example, requires activated sulfate in the form of 3'-phosphoadenosine 5'-phosphosulfate (PAPS). Further, sulfate is added to the completed carbohydrate chains rather than to free monomers. Glycoprotein synthesis is dependent on the nature of the linkage between the carbohydrate and protein. For those glycoproteins where the link is between asparagine and N-acetylglucosamine, the carobhydrate chain is formed on a lipid carrier, dolichoyl phosphate, and then transferred to protein. If the link is between a carbohydrate and serine or threonine, however, no lipid intermediate is involved and the monomers are added sequentially to the protein.

REVIEW QUESTIONS

1. What is the general process for formation of starch and glycogen?
2. What is dolichol phosphate?
3. How do the syntheses of asparagine-linked and serine-linked glycoproteins differ?
4. Where are mucopolysaccharides primarily degraded?

BIBLIOGRAPHY

Adair, W., and Keller, R.   1982.   Dolichol metabolism in rat liver. J. Biol. Chem. *257*, 8990–8996.

Bunn, H., and Higgins, P.   1981.   Reaction of monosaccharides with proteins: possible evolutionary significance. Science *213*, 222–224.

Carson, D., and Lennarz, W.   1981.   Relationship of dolichol synthesis to glycoprotein synthesis during embryonic development. J. Biol. Chem. *256*, 4679–4686.

Carson, D., Earles, B., and Lennarz, W.   1981.   Enhancement of protein glycosylation in tissue slices by dolicholphosphate. J. Biol. Chem. *256*, 11552–11557.

Elbein, A.   1981.   The tunicamycins—useful tools for studies on glycoproteins. Trends Biochem. Sci. *6*, 219–221.

Gershman, H., and Robbins, P.   1981.   Transitory effects of glucose starvation on the synthesis of dolichol-linked oligosaccharides in mammalian cells. J. Biol. Chem. *256*, 7774–7780.

Harrison, F., and Chesterton, C.   1980.   Factors mediating cell-cell recognition and adhesion. FEBS Lett. *122*, 157–164.

Horowitz, M. and Pigman, W. (Editors).   1982.   The Glycoconjugates, Vol. 3, Glycoproteins, Glycolipids and Proteoglycans. Academic Press, New York.

Hughes, R., and Butters, T.   1981.   Glycosylation patterns in cells: an evolutionary marker. Trends Biochem. Sci. *6*, 228–230.

Jaques, L.   1979.   Forty years of heparin research—past and future. *In* Heparin: Structure, Cellular Functions and Clinical Applications. N. McDuffie (Editor). Academic Press, New York.

Jenkins, R., Hall, T., and Dorfman, A.   1981.   Chondroitin 6-sulfate oligosaccharide as immunological determinants of chick proteoglycans. J. Biol. Chem. *256*, 8279–8282.

Keller, R., Jehle, E., and Adair, W.   1982.   The origin of dolichol in the liver of the rat. J. Biol. Chem. *257*, 8985–8989.

Murphy, L., and Spiro, R.   1981.   Transfer of glucose to oligosaccharide-lipid intermediates by thyroid microsomal enzymes and its relationship to the N-glycosylation of proteins. J. Biol. Chem. *256*, 7487–7794.

Nikaido, H., and Hassid, W.   1971.   Biosynthesis of saccharides from glycopyranosyl esters of nucleoside pyrophosphates ("sugar nucleotides"). Adv. Carbohydr. Chem. Biochem. *26*, 351–483.

Pierce, J., and Parsons, T.   1981.   Glycoprotein hormones: structure and function. Annu. Rev. Biochem. *50*, 465–495.

Riesenfeld, J., Hook, M., and Lindahl, U.   1982.   Biosynthesis of heparin. J. Biol. Chem. *257*, 421–425.

Rome, L., and Crain, L.   1981.   Degradation of mucopolysaccharides in isolated intact lysosomes. J. Biol. Chem. *256*, 10763–10768.

Schachter, H., Narasimhan, S., and Wilson, J.   1978.   Biosynthesis and catabolism of glycoproteins. *In* Glycoproteins and Glycolipids in Disease Processes. Am. Chem. Soc., Washington, D.C.

Sell, S.   1978.   Alpha-fetoprotein as an indicator of early events in chemical carcinogenesis. *In* Glycoproteins and Glycolipids in Diseases Processes. Am. Chem. Soc., Washington, D.C.

Staneloni, R., and Leloir, L.   1982.   The biosynthetic pathway of the asparagine-linked oligosaccharides of glycoproteins. CRC Crit. Rev. Biochem. *12*, 289–326.

Stevens, R., Nessley, S., Kimura, J., Rechler, M., Caplan, A., and Hascall, V.   1981.   Effects of insulin and multiplication-stimulating activity on proteoglycan biosynthesis in chondrocytes from the swarm rat chondrosarcoma. J. Biol. Chem. *256*, 2045–2052.

Wagh, P., and Bahl, O.   1981.   Sugar residues on proteins. CRC Crit. Rev. Biochem. *10*, 307–377.

11

Hormonal Effects on Carbohydrate Metabolism

A. INTRODUCTION

Carbohydrate metabolism (both synthesis and degration) is highly subject to the hormonal influences on the cell. A variety of hormones, including insulin, glucagon, catecholamines, glucocorticoids, thyroid hormone, and growth hormone, all can profoundly influence the course of carbohydrate metabolism. Sometimes the hormones act synergistically and sometimes in opposition. Their effects may be enhanced, blunted, or mediated by other factors as well. In general, carbohydrate is stored during periods of "plenty." When calories are consumed in excess of immediate requirements, then the surplus can be stored. The storage of carbohydrate may take several forms: carbohydrate can be stored as a carbohydrate polymer (glycogen) or it can be converted into fat and stored for periods when food is not available. Storage of carbohydrate as glycogen has several advantages. Only a few enzymatic steps are involved in making glycogen from glucose so there are few places for errors to occur. When glucose is stored as glycogen, it can be easily reconverted to glucose for release to the bloodstream. A disadvantage of glycogen storage is that there is considerable hydration involved (about 4 g water for each gram of glycogen). Thus, the animal must carry considerable extra weight with its fuel supply. Fat, on the other hand, is more calorically dense (9 kcal/g fat vs. 4 kcal/g carbohydrate) and is not hydrated. Therefore, many more "calories" of fuel can be maintained at a far lower weight. Fatty acids, however, cannot be converted to glucose although the glycerol portion can. Thus, fat is not a ready source of glucose like glycogen. If fat is the primary fuel then glucose must be supplied at the expense of body protein stores.

There is an ordered entry of fuels into various stores. Glycogen stores are repleted first, which attests to the importance of these stores to body function. After the glycogen stores are well filled, then fat is rapidly produced from any excess dietary carbohydrate.

When an animal has been fasted for a time and then is refed, glycogen stores are refilled to greater than normal levels. In a sense, the animal is "making up for lost time." Under ordinary conditions in the wild, food is often scarce and food supplies are unpredictable. If an animal could replete body stores only at the same rate at which they were lost, it is easy to see that the animal would soon dwindle and die. If, on the other hand, an animal can readily take advantage of available food to rebuild body stores at a rapid rate, then it will be able to cope with the next period of scarce food. Should you fail to believe this, take note the next time you are ill and cannot eat. Note your rapid weight loss. "Wow, I'm well on my way to getting rid of those unwanted pounds," you say. Then you feel better and start to eat. The pounds come back almost immediately. This repletion device, which is ultimately hormonally controlled, is fine protection for animals in conditions where food is sparse. It tends, however, to work against the well-fed person in our modern society.

The distribution of endogenously stored nutrients is (and needs to be) under the influence of several hormones because there are a variety of different circumstances under which these stored nutrients are required. For example, a fasting man at rest has different needs than a fed man engaged in vigorous physical activity. Needs are both short and long term. The thyroid hormones regulate long-term metabolic efficiency whereas the catecholomines influence short-term events. Insulin and glucagon are critical in the day-to-day homeostasis of blood glucose, but glucocorticoids and thyroid hormone provide that extra moderating influence required during periods of stress. These are but a few of the interacting factors. Loss of regulation by any one of the hormones (e.g., insulin in diabetes) may not result in the death of the organism, but it does seriously impair the ability of that organism to function optimally under the variety of physiological conditions and environmental stresses normally encountered.

B. INSULIN AND GLUCAGON

The two hormones, insulin and glucagon, shall be considered together since they are opposite sides of the same coin. What has come to be known as the Sherringtonian metaphor is operative in most hormonal situations. Initially Sherrington applied the idea of opposing forces to muscles. That is, one muscle always works against another and not against free space. Such is the case with normal insulin and glucagon release and function. When blood glucose levels rise, insulin is released resulting in a drop in blood glucose. This decrease does not occur indefinitely, however, as it might if there were no opposing force. Instead when the level of blood glucose reaches a critical level, glucagon is released triggering the pathways that contribute glucose to the bloodstream. This sort of seesaw in insulin and glucagon results in a cyclical rise and fall of blood glucose within rather narrowly defined limits. If only one hormone were involved, the oscillations in blood glucose would be far larger, perhaps with serious consequences for the animal.

Let us examine the release and function of these hormones. Insulin is released from the β cells of the pancreas. These cells are found in the islet tissue, which is concentrated in the tail of the pancreas and comprises 1–2% of the weight of the total pancreas. The β cells are round with a crystalline structure. The islets are interposed around heavy networks of capillaries and are highly innervated, which is to be expected since the islet cells are in intimate connection with the rest of the body.

Although the releasing mechanism for insulin is not yet completely clear, it is much better understood than the action of insulin on target cells. After a carbohydrate rich meal, 70% of the glucose in portal blood is retained by liver. However, there is sufficient rise in serum glucose to trigger release of insulin from the β cell. Further, the prepriming devices in the gut, most notably gastric inhibitory polypeptide, also enhance insulin release.

Insulin release occurs within seconds after serum glucose begins to rise. The magnitude of the initial insulin release is proportional to the glucose concentration over a wide range of glucose levels. The initial rise in insulin secretion is quickly followed by a return to near basal levels and next by a slower, sustained rise in insulin secretion which is maintained as long as the glucose stimulus is present (Fig. 11.1). The initial rise in insulin is called Phase I release and the sustained, secondary rise is called Phase II release. The two phases have some similarities and differences. Puromycin, a protein synthesis inhibitor, has no effect on Phase I and a partial inhibitory effect on Phase II. Tolbutamide, an oral hypoglycemic agent used to stimulate insulin release in diabetics, affects Phase I but not Phase II. On the other hand, both phases obligatorily require extracellular calcium. No new β granule formation is observed in Phase I but there is in Phase II. Both phases are inhibited by oligomycin which indicates that insulin release is an energy requiring process. Experiments with leucine pulse labeling suggest that the first insulin made is the first secreted. It is also fairly

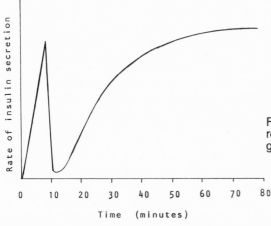

FIG. 11.1 Biphasic insulin release in response to a glucose stimulus.

certain that the initial spike is not due to insulin inhibition of further secretion. Secretion of insulin can occur in either phase only when the glucose concentration is in excess of 50 mg/dl.

Several models for insulin release have been proposed (Chan and Steiner 1977). The first is the two compartment model, which states that there is a small compartment with rapid kinetics which accounts for Phase I release and a large compartment with slow kinetics accounting for Phase II. Although this model is initially satisfying it does not successfully explain all the available data. The multiplicative model better fits the data. This model states that glucose at the β cell triggers three events with different time courses: initiation of insulin release, potentiation of synthesis, and negative feedback on insulin release. More work is needed to definitively adopt this model.

The process of insulin synthesis and secretion can be visualized as follows. The initiating event occurs when glucose attaches to a β cell receptor causing uptake of extracellular calcium. In the absence of extracellular calcium, release does not occur. If glucose levels are too low (less than 50 mg/dl) then release again cannot occur. This amounts to a double protection mechanism insuring that conditions are just right before insulin is allowed to be released. A general scheme of insulin manufacture and release is shown in Fig. 11.2. As the result of interaction of glucose with the glucose receptor on the surface of the β cell, there is initiation of preproinsulin synthesis. The protein precursor is clipped to form proinsulin (an energy requiring process), which becomes associated with the Golgi apparatus. A further proteolytic clip is made yielding insulin and C peptide. The β granules are then formed. By the time they reach the cytoplasm, they will be ready to take up Zn^{2+} to form crystalline Zn-insulin inside the granules. The β granules then become associated with the microtubules and in an apparent peristaltic-like process are pushed toward the cell membrane. Under an appropriate stimulus, the β granules fuse with the cellular membrane, rupture, and extrude their contents out of the β cell. Equal quantities of native insulin and C peptide are released into the bloodstream. With one exception (calcium ionophores), blood glucose levels must be higher than 40–50 mg% in order for insulin to be released. This has led to two schools of thought concerning the role of glucose in insulin release. One theory suggests that the act of glucose binding to a pancreatic receptor is sufficient to trigger release. The second proposal requires that glucose be metabolized and that a metabolite is the actual trigger for insulin release. A number of intermediates have been suggested for this role including glucose 1,6-bisphosphate and fructose 2,6-bisphosphate. Presently, neither mechanism can be confirmed.

The percentage of proinsulin in the pancreas is 2–9% but in the plasma it is slightly higher because it is metabolized more slowly. Preproinsulin was discovered in 1976. Because of its extremely rapid turnover, it is nearly transparent to labeling studies. In this molecule there is a 2500 dalton extension on the amino terminal end consisting

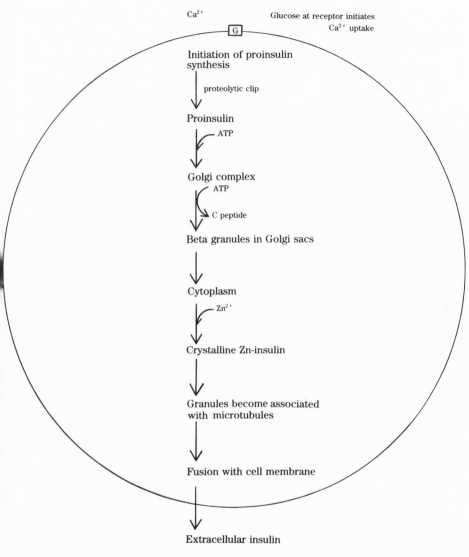

FIG. 11.2.   General scheme of insulin synthesis and release from pancreatic B cells.

of many hydrophobic side chains. This amino terminal chain is fairly typical of most proteins made for export and may be necessary for proper membrane binding to allow extrusion from the cell.

The Golgi, microtubules, and microfilaments are very important to the processing and export of proteins such as insulin. An interesting review of Golgi structure and function has recently appeared (Rothman 1981). This organelle provides the processing and sorting of the insulin molecules. The microtubules are composed of proteins similar to actin and provide a route for export of insulin. Microfilaments, on the other hand, are smaller and are composed of single filaments, which may act as a barrier to the fusion of the cellular membrane around the β granules. Cytochalasin B disrupts microfilaments but does not harm microtubules. As would be expected, cytochalasin B results in a two- to threefold increase in Phase I insulin secretion similar to the effect of tolbutamide. Cholchicine, on the other hand, disrupts microtubules and therefore decreases insulin release.

Cyclic AMP also seems to be involved in insulin release but its exact mechanism of action remains unknown. When exogenous cyclic AMP or agents which elevate cyclic AMP are added to islets, insulin release is stimulated only in the presence of elevated glucose. Serum D-glucose does raise cyclic AMP levels in islets but not in adipose tissue. There are several hypotheses for how this might come about: there could be direct stimulation of adenylate cyclase, or enlargement of a specific ATP pool serving as substrate for adenylate cyclase or inhibition of phosphodiesterase. The rise in cyclic AMP could be coincident rather than causal. That is, it could be the result of glucose dependent translocation of calcium. Indeed, calcium does activate a calmodulin sensitive adenylate cyclase. Glucose does cause a net flux of Ca^{2+} from extra- to intracellular space, and diazoxide, which in a potent inhibitor of insulin release, also inhibits calcium induced insulin release.

The only compound that will release insulin in the absence of glucose is the ionophore A23187. Theophylline, a methyl xanthine in the same family as caffeine, also stimulates insulin release and may do so by altering calcium levels. Tolbutamide's mechanism of action is as yet unknown. Alloxan damages the β cell, but the effect is blocked by glucose or 3-O-methylglucose. Epinephrine blocks insulin release by α-adrenergic receptors, which are also believed to be coupled in some way with calcium flux. The structural similarities of the compounds can be observed by examining Fig. 11.3.

Less is known about glucagon release but it is believed that it is a good bit like insulin release. It is known that there is a 65,000 MW immunoreactive glucagon precursor that is clipped to progulcagon which is devoid of hormonal activity. Progulcagon is further reduced in size to a 4000 MW polypeptide and finally to true glucagon. Glucagon secretion is blocked by insulin secretion. The secretion of both glucagon and insulin as well as a number of other hormones is blocked by the 14 amino acid release-inhibiting hormone, somatostatin. The physiological role of somatostatin still needs clarification.

In order to exert effects at the cellular level, glucagon and insulin must travel through the serum and bind to specific receptors on target cells. It seems clear that the receptor for glucagon is coupled in some way to adenylate cyclase located in the plasma membrane and that all the actions of glucagon are mediated through cyclic AMP. The couple

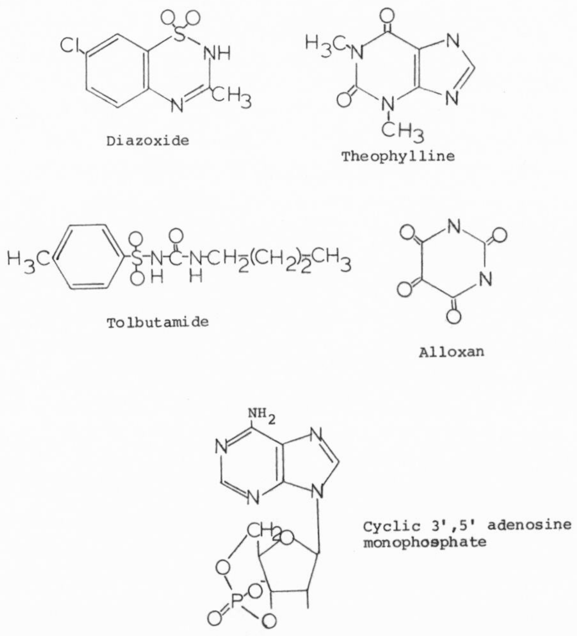

Diazoxide

Theophylline

Tolbutamide

Alloxan

Cyclic 3',5' adenosine monophosphate

FIG. 11.3. Compounds altering insulin secretion.

between glucagon and this enzyme may not be direct and there may be a membrane bound coupling molecule(s) between the actual receptor and the enzyme. Adenylate cyclase also has a high affinity nucleotide site specific for GTP which activates the enzyme. This site may not be important in all hormone stimulation of the enzyme, but it is obligatory in catecholamine stimulation. Adenylate cyclase is relatively large (~200,000 MW) and is activated by fluoride ion and must be membrane bound to be hormone sensitive.

Glucagon activation of adenylate cyclase is very rapid (steady state after 10 sec) and can be reversed within 1 min or so. Only about 10% of the glucagon receptors on the cell surface have to be occupied in order to get a maximum stimulation of the enzyme. Cyclic AMP levels begin to rise when adenylate cyclase is activated. The cyclic AMP then binds to the regulatory subunits of cyclic AMP dependent protein kinase liberating the free, active catalytic subunits. The stoichiometry for this is

$$R_2C_2 + 4 \text{ cAMP} \dashrightarrow 2 R-4 \text{ cAMP} + 2 C$$

A protease specific for the free catalytic subunit has been isolated (Alhanaty and Shaltiel 1979) which may be important in regulating the quantity of catalytic subunit available to phosphorylate other proteins. The catalytic subunit phosphorylates susceptible proteins with the γ-phosphate from ATP. In general, enzymes involved in fuel break-down are activated by this phosphorylation whereas those which are involved with fuel storage are inactivated. Glucagon, therefore, acti-vates the enzymes associated with glycogen breakdown and inacti-vates those resulting in glycogen and fat synthesis.

Insulin interaction with the receptor is less well understood. For years it was believed that insulin could only function as the result of binding to cell surface receptors. More recently evidence has been pre-sented that insulin is rapidly internalized. There may be some recy-cling of the insulin receptor back to the cell surface under some condi-tions. Since insulin is rapidly inactivated, it is quite possible that the internalization is a degradative process and not part of the mechanism whereby insulin alters cellular activities. Recently, it has been re-ported (Jarrett and Seals, 1979; Larner *et al.*, 1979) that insulin bind-ing to its receptor promotes the release of a small molecule that then acts as the second messenger for insulin inside the cell. Although it is logical to assume that insulin should function by stimulating phos-phatases, data are not yet available to support so sweeping an assump-tion. Insulin does promote fuel storage and inhibit fuel breakdown. Other mechanisms of action have been suggested. One potential mech-anism is the stimulation of ion (probably calcium) fluxes in the cell. It is known that insulin can indeed alter the subcellular distribution of calcium (McDonald *et al.* 1976). Other potential models have been discussed by Czech (1977) and include such other mechanisms as cyclic nucleotide dependent phosphorylation, transmembrane potentials, monovalent cation flux, the thiol redox model, and phospholipid turnover.

Rather more is known about the nature of the insulin receptor per se. The receptor may consist of two separate types of receptors or a single receptor having two independent functions. For example, many cells require insulin for glucose entry whereas other cells (e.g., liver and brain) do not. Even cells that do not require insulin for glucose entry may still have their metabolic events profoundly influenced by insulin. Available evidence suggests that insulin effect on glucose en-try is a separate function with very rapid kinetics whereas influence on metabolic events is another function. In adipose tissue, insulin seems to increase the number of functional glucose transporters.

The number of insulin receptors ranges from 2000 per cell in human erythrocytes to 300,000 per cell in human adipocytes. The affinities (k_a) of receptors range from 0.01 nM for erythrocytes to 1.6 nM for adipocytes. The receptor is highly specific for insulin and does not bind other polypeptide hormones such as glucagon. Once the insulin recep-tors are solubilized from their respective membranes, the similarities are striking regardless of their tissue or species of origin. They weigh about 300,000 daltons, have a Stokes radius of ~70 Å, and are asym-metric proteins. They are probably glycoproteins as are many cell sur-face proteins. Czech and his colleagues (1981) have proposed an $(\alpha\beta)_2$

subunit structure for intact adipocyte receptors. The subunits are apparently connected by disulfide bonds. Using affinity labeling of isolated plasma membrane these workers found a $\alpha\beta$ and $\alpha\beta_1$ subunit structure where β was quite similar in structure to β_1. They concluded, however, that β_1 was generated from β by limited proteolysis and that the intact, native structure was indeed $(\alpha\beta)_2$.

Regulation of the number of insulin receptors on the cell surface may have a profound effect on the ability of insulin to influence cellular events. When serum insulin concentrations are high, the number of receptors may be diminished. In effect, this limits the sensitivity of the cell to the hormone and protects the cell against overstimulation. This phenomenon, known as down regulation, is not unique to insulin receptors but rather appears to apply to a variety of hormone receptors. There is some evidence that the receptors are "swallowed" by the cell and that they may be returned to the cell surface when a change in the extracellular environment warrants. Receptor turnover and processing and its relationship to metabolic control promise to be some of the most fascinating areas of future research.

C. CATECHOLAMINES

The catecholamines, epinephrine and norepinephrine, impinge on carbohydrate metabolism in a number of different ways. First, the pancreas is highly innervated, and the islet tissue has contact with adrenergic as well as cholinergic axon terminals. Norepinephrine influences the β cell via two receptors and therefore has several different effects on this cell. If the interaction occurs via the α receptor, insulin secretion is diminished both basally and in response to glucose. Interaction through the β receptor, however, leads to enhanced insulin release. Although this may appear conflicting, it offers a considerable regulatory advantage during periods of short-term stress. A further regulatory influence is also available at the pancreatic level because catecholamines stimulate glucagon secretion via the β receptor. Although there may be some catecholamine α receptor interaction, it is thought to be relatively unimportant to the overall regulation of the α cell.

Catecholamines can alter carbohydrate metabolism at the target cell level as well. In the liver cell, most of the interaction of catecholamines is mediated through the α receptors. These receptors are not coupled to the adenylate cyclase–cyclic AMP–protein kinase system of control. Instead, the effects of catecholamines are mediated through calcium ion flux out of the mitochondria (and perhaps the endoplasmic reticulum) into the cytoplasm. The increased calcium level stimulates enzymes such as phosphorylase kinase, the initial step in the glycogen degradation cascade. Thus, an animal who becomes frightened secretes epinephrine into the circulation, some of which binds to liver cells. As a result, glycogen synthesis is turned off and glycogen degradation is stimulated, providing glucose for the bloodstream. In this case, fat synthesis also declines because it would be unfortunate indeed if the glucose produced which was destined for the bloodstream was instead turned into fat. Since there are no α receptors on the mitochondria and studies with immobilized epinephrine indicate that epinephrine does not need to enter the mitochondria to function, there must be some sort of second messenger generated to communicate receptor binding to the mitochondrial calcium pool. The identity of this messenger is still a secret of nature.

In contrast to liver, epinephrine effects on muscle occur via the β receptor. Studies from Exton's laboratory (Shikama *et al.* 1981) have indicated that insulin activation of glycogen synthetase is reversed by epinephrine. Insulin, however, does not change the cyclic AMP concentration or the activity of protein kinase. From a physiological standpoint, these interactions make a great deal of sense. The muscles of a frightened animal must be metabolically poised to prepare it for flight. This requires that any insulin effect be overridden. The opposite case would be undesirable: one would wish epinephrine to take precedence over insulin at the muscle regardless of the serum insulin levels or the dietary state of the animal. An animal who successfully escapes a predator can live to eat for another day.

There may be one other interaction in the insulin/catecholamine tug-of-war, which is important to the diabetic receiving sulfonylurea-type drugs. It may be that sulfonylureas not only stimulate insulin release from the β cell but also inhibit catecholamine release from the adrenal gland. Since some cases of diabetes could result from or be aggravated by excess production of counterregulatory hormones, then it seems likely that the sulfonylurea hypolycemic agents may function in part to reduce the antagonism of insulin function by such counterregulatory agents as catecholamines.

D. GLUCOCORTICOIDS

The primary function of glucocorticoids is to protect against stress, especially in the long term. It has been suggested that one reason that women are less susceptible than men to stress related illnesses is that they have higher levels of glucocorticoids. Glucocorticoids have generally been considered to be "permissive" rather than direct hormonal effectors. This idea has over the years become modified to include a direct hormonal action, which may not be immediately expressed but which is crucial to the metabolic adjustments the organism must make under various environmental conditions.

In general, the function of the glucocorticoids is to make fuel more readily available for times of need. An adrenalectomized animal, for example, readily survives with a constant food supply but dies after several hours if food is unavailable. In the presence of glucocorticoids, proteins and fats are broken down as the result of enhanced gluconeogenesis and lipolysis, respectively, whereas glycogen storage is enhanced. This is in contrast to the action of epinephrine which increases gluconeogenesis and lipolysis as well as glycogenolysis. If glucocorticoids are absent as the result of adrenalectomy, then the animal cannot provide blood glucose via gluconeogenesis and energy via the breakdown of fat.

Glucocorticoids are synthesized in the zona fasiculata and to a lesser extent in the zona reticularis of the adrenal cortex (Fig. 11.4). In order for glucocorticoids to be released from the cortex, there must first be stimulation of the cortex by adrenalcorticotropin (ACTH) which is a 4500 MW peptide released from the pituitary in response to corticotropin releasing factor (CRF) from the hypothalamus. ACTH acts at the cell surface (probably through cyclic AMP) to stimulate the rate limiting step in glucocorticoid synthesis. This step is between cholesterol and progresterone, occurs in the mitchondria, and requires NADPH and O_2.

Cortisol is the glucocorticoid produced in the highest concentration in man and corticosterone is the most prevalent in rats. After leaving the adrenal, glucocorticoids are transported in the serum on transcortin (corticoid binding globulin), a protein with a very high affinity for glucocorticoids.

At the cellular level, the glucocorticoid receptor is apparently a bit different from the receptors for insulin and glucagon. There are about 5000–10,000 sites per cell but the sites are not on the plasma membrane. The glucocorticoids bind to a cytoplasmic receptor to form a complex; this is the rate-limiting step. The complex is then translocated to the nucleus where it seems to function by altering the cell's

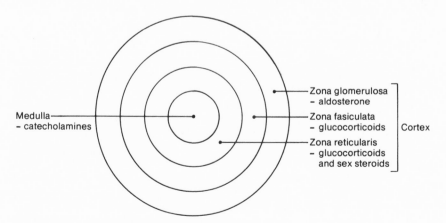

FIG. 11.4. Products of the adrenal gland.

TABLE 11.1.   Cellular Glucocorticoid Binders

Form	MW	Function
Binder I (ligandin)	40,000	Nonspecific binding of a number of compounds
Binder II	67,000	Pysiological receptor
Binder III	7,000	Degradative form, binds preferentially to monosulfated form of glucocorticoid. Contains nucleotides
Binder IV	50,000–60,000	Contains transcortin

protein synthetic machinery. Actually, there are four proteins in the cyloplasm which bind glucocorticoids with high affinity. Their properties are shown in Table 11.1.

E. GROWTH HORMONE (SOMATOTROPIN)

Growth hormone (~22,000 MW) has a number of actions, some of which seem to be conflicting at first glance. This hormone stimulates amino acid uptake and protein synthesis, lipolysis and gluconeogenesis from lactate, and glycogenolysis. In some respects, somatotropin is like insulin and in others it is like the glucocorticoids. One may tend to think of this hormone being important only in the preadult stages of life. In view of the fact that growth hormone levels remain high throughout adult life even though growth has ceased, it is likely that this hormone continues to play an important role in metabolism. It is likely that its main functions are to maintain blood glucose levels and to protect against massive tissue destruction during fasting.

Since growth hormone is also released during stress, it acts synergistically with glucocorticoids. With regard to lipolysis these hormones function in the same direction but counteract each other on gluconeogenesis and glycogenolysis. This allows for a much more controlled regulatory climate than would be the case with a single hormone. Overdoses of growth hormone lead to a pseudo-diabetic state called idiohypophysial diabetes. The result is hyperglycemia and visceral fat deposition with peripheral fat depletion.

The mechanism of action of growth hormone at the cellular level is not clear. Most cells, however, are sensitive to the hormone. Even though the effects of the hormone are delayed, interaction of the cell with the hormone for periods of less than 1 min can result in triggered reactions at a subsequent time. Early on, cellular glucose uptake is enhanced and later it is diminished. The reasons for this behavior are not clear. It might be postulated that the time delay represents the time for a second messenger to form. Although in some cases, growth hormone may precipitate a rise in cyclic AMP, this does not always occur, and it is doubtful that cyclic AMP is the true messenger for this hormone.

E. OTHER HORMONAL EFFECTS

A number of other hormones can also influence carbohydrate metabolism. Important among these are the female sex hormones. Alterations of carbohydrate metabolism are frequently observed during pregnancy and often during oral contraceptive use. Both progestagens and estrogens are involved. Abnormal glucose tolerance tests are frequently noted although frank diabetes is not common.

Other hormonal effects include those that alter feeding behavior. The hypothalamus is an important site of satiety and appetite regulation. Not only does this organ affect food intake but surgically causing lesions in it prevents or causes the loss of feeding behavior. These surgically altered animals, however, are not just normal animals without an appetite. They lose relatively more protein stores and less fat than a normal fasted animal. One of the hormones that may be involved in feeding regulation is cholecystokinin, which is released in response to feeding. Infusion of cholecystokinin into the hypothalamic region stops feeding behavior. It has also been noted that there is less cholecystokinin in the brains of obese animals compared to lean controls (Straus and Yalow 1979).

Thyroid hormone, which is responsible for setting metabolic rate (or metabolic efficiency), can also have profound consequences on carbohydrate metabolism. The process leading to the release of thyroid hormone is outlined in Fig. 11.5. Like glucocorticoids, T_3 and T_4 are said to be "permissive" but undoubtedly their actions are direct but long term. Thyroid hormones at high levels cause lipolysis, gluconeogenesis, and glycogenolysis and blood glucose levels become elevated. The mechanisms of these effects, like those of so many other hormones, remain unknown.

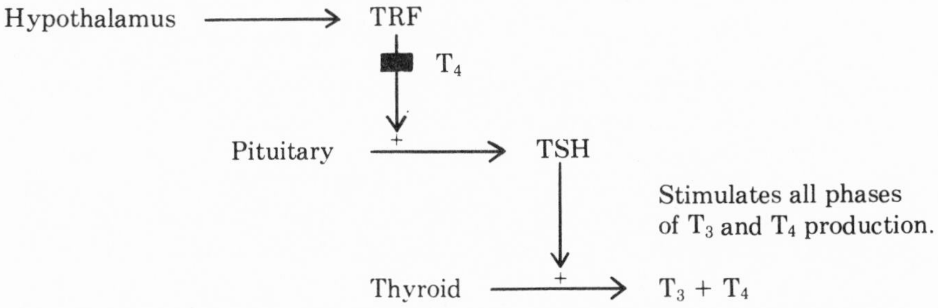

Hypothalamus $\longrightarrow$ TRF

$\downarrow$ T_4

Pituitary $\xrightarrow{\quad + \quad}$ TSH

Stimulates all phases of T_3 and T_4 production.

Thyroid $\xrightarrow{\quad + \quad}$ $T_3 + T_4$

FIG. 11.5. Release of thyroid hormone. TRF, thyroid releasing factor: Glu-His-Pro (same in all species). TSH, thyroid stimulating hormone: 25,000 MW glycoprotein.

G. SUMMARY

The regulation of carbohydrate metabolism depends on a number of hormones. Short-term effects are brought about by such hormones as insulin, glucagon, and catecholamines. Longer term effects are mediated by glucocorticoids, thyroid hormone, growth hormone, and others such as estrogen. All hormones must work via a cellular receptor but not all receptors are alike. Some may be typical of the glucagon receptor, which is a cell membrane protein coupled in some way to adenylate cyclase. Alternatively, some may be similar to the α receptor for catecholamines which, when stimulated, causes an ion flux between various cellular compartments. Another possibility is the mobile receptor complex similar to that for glucocorticoids where the hormones after entering the cell, bind to an internal receptor, and are then carried to their site(s) of action. The regulation of receptor quantity may also be an important control over the relationship between a hormone and a target cell. When hormone levels become very high, a cell can protect itself by reducing the number of receptors for that hormone. The hormones that affect carbohydrate metabolism may function in concert or in opposition or at some level in between. This wide range of effects provides a much more "finely tuned" environment and better enables an animal to adapt to environmental changes.

REVIEW QUESTIONS

1. In liver, which receptor mediates catecholamine effects?
2. Describe the physiological glucocorticoid binder?
3. What are the characteristics of the insulin receptor?
4. What are the effects of insulin, glucagon, and glucococorticoids on gluconeogenesis, lipolysis, and glycogen degradation?

BIBLIOGRAPHY

Alhanaty, E., and Shaltiel, S.   1979.   Limited proteolysis of the catalytic subunit of c-AMP dependent protein kinase—a membrane regulatory device. Biochem. Biophys. Res. Commun. 89, 323–332.

Baxter, J., and Rousseau, G.   1979.   Glucocorticoid Hormone Action. Springer-Verlag, New York.

Brownlee, M.   1981.   Handbook of Diabetes Mellitus, Vol. II. Garland STPM Press, New York.

Caro, J., and Amaturda, J.   1980.   Insulin receptors in hepatocytes: post receptor events mediate down regulation. Science 210, 1029–1031.

Chan, S., and Steiner, D.   1977.   Pre-proinsulin, a new precursor in insulin biosynthesis. Trends Biochem. Sci. 2, 254–256.

Corin, R., and Donner, D.   1981.   Up regulation of insulin receptors in rat liver plasma membranes. J. Biol. Chem. 256, 11413–11416.

Czech, M.   1977.   Insulin action. Annu. Rev. Biochem. 46, 359–384.

Czech, M., Massague, J., and Pilch, P.   1981.   The insulin receptor: structural features. Trends Biochem. Sci. 6, 222–225.

Gliemann, J., and Sönne, O. 1977. The mechanism of action of polypeptide hormones with special reference to insulin's action on glucose transport. Clin. Endocrinal. 7, 405–415.

Goldfine, I. 1978. Insulin receptors and the site of action of insulin. Life Sci. 23, 2639–2648.

Grodsky, G., Sando, H., Levin, S., Gerich, J., and Karam, J. 1977. Synthesis and secretion of insulin in dynamic perfusion systems. Adv. Metab. Disorders 7, 155–170.

Jarett, L., and Seals, J. 1979. Pyruvate dehydrogenase activation in adipocyte mitochondria by an insulin generated mediator from muscle. Science 206, 1407–1408.

Karnieli, E., Zarnowski, M., Hissin, P., Simpson, I., Salans, L., and Cushman, S. 1981. Insulin stimulated translocation of glucose transport systems in the isolated rat adipose cell. J. Biol. Chem. 256, 4772–4777.

Larner, J., Galasko, G., Cheng, K., DePaoli-Roach, A., Huang, L., Daggy, P., and Kellogg, J. 1979. Generation of a chemical mediator that controls protein phosphorylation and dephosphorylation. Science 206, 1408–1410.

Ludvigsen, C., and Jarett, L. 1982. Simularities between hydrogen peroxide, concanavalin A and anti-insulin receptor antibody stimulated glucose transport: increase in the number of transport sites. Metabolism 31, 284–287.

McDonald, J., Bruns, D., and Jarett, L. 1976. The ability of insulin to alter the stable calcium pools of isolated adipocyte subcellular fractions. Biochem. Biophys. Res. Commun. 71, 114–121.

Marshall, S., Green, A., and Olefsky, J. 1981. Evidence for recycling of insulin receptors in isolated rat adipocytes. J. Biol. Chem. 256, 11464–11470.

Montague, W. 1979. Cyclic nucleotides, calcium and insulin secretion. In Cyclic 3',5' Nucleotides: Mechanisms of Action. H. Cramer and J. Schultz (Editors). J. Wiley & Sons, New York.

Pilch, P., and Czech, M. 1980. Hormone binding alters the conforation of the insulin receptor. Science 210, 1152–1153.

Plas, C., and Desbuquois, B. 1982. Receptor mediated insulin degradation and insulin stimulated glycogenesis in cultured fetal hepatocytes. Biochem. J. 202, 333–341.

Posner, B., Patel, B., Khan, M., and Bergeron, J. 1982. Effect of chloroquine on the internalization of ^{125}I-insulin into subcellular fractions of rat liver. J. Biol. Chem. 257, 5789–5799.

Rasmussen, H., and Waisman, D. 1981. The messenger function of calcium in endocrine systems. In Biochemical Actions of Hormones, Vol. VIII. G. Litwack (Editor). Academic Press, New York.

Rothman, J. 1981. The golgi. Science 213, 1212–1219.

Sener, A., Malaisse-Lagae, F., and Malaisse, W. 1982. Glucose-induced accumulation of glucose 1,6-bisphosphate in pancreatic islets: its possible role in the regulation of glycolysis. Biochem. Biophys. Res.Commun. 104, 1033–1040.

Shikama, H., Chaisson, J., and Exton, J. 1981. Studies on the interactions between insulin and epinephrine in the control of skeletal muscle glycogen metabolism. J. Biol. Chem. 256, 4450–4454.

Straus, E., and Yalow, R. 1979. Cholecystokinin in the brains of obese and non-obese mice. Science 203, 68–69.

Suzuki, K., and Kono, T. 1979. Internalization and degradation of fat cell bound insulin. Separation and partial characterization of subcellular vesicles associated with iodoinsulin. J. Biol. Chem. 254, 9786–9794.

Tepperman, J., and Tepperman, H. 1958. Effects of antecedent food intake patterns on hepatic lipogenesis. Am. J. Physiol. 193, 55–64.

Part **IV**

Disorders of Carbohydrate Metabolism

12

Diabetes

A. TYPES AND FREQUENCY

Diabetes mellitus is the inability to maintain blood glucose home-ostasis, and the levels of blood glucose are inappropriately high. A victim of this disease may experience polyphagia, polydypsia, and polyuria. Diabetes mellitus was first described in an ancient Egyptian papyrus. In the United States approximately one of every five people will ultimately have diabetes, and the risk of becoming a diabetic increases with age. Although there is some natural deterioration of glucose tolerance as one ages, which is unrelated to diabetes, correct-ing for this still leaves a proportionately higher percentage of the disease among the elderly in the population. The impairment that begins in the third or fourth decade of life is due to tissue unrespon-siveness to insulin while insulin release from the pancreas in response to glucose remains normal.

The earlier literature defined essentially two main types of diabetes. These were the juvenile and adult-onset types. Characteristics of each type are shown in Table 12.1. The American Diabetes Association has now recommended that the names of the two types be altered to re-move some of the ambiguity in the criteria for each type. The new classifications are "insulin-dependent diabetes" (Type I), which corre-sponds approximately to the juvenile type, and "insulin-independent diabetes" (Type II), which corresponds roughly to the adult-onset type. Type III, formerly called secondary diabetes, is the result of some other disease or syndrome such as accidental pancreatic damage. This new

TABLE 12.1.   Characteristics of Juvenile and Adult-Onset Diabetes

Characteristics	Juvenile	Adult-onset
Age	Young	Middle-aged
Weight	Normal	Overweight
Ketoacidosis	Frequent	Seldom
Serum insulin levels	Low	Normal to high
Effect of stress	Complicates treatment	Little effect
Complications	Widely fluctuating blood glucose levels	Hyperglycemia leading to a coma

classification allows for a better distinction of the phenomenon of adult-onset diabetic who become insulin dependent.

In terms of genetic correlation, it is easier to establish genetic links in adult-onset diabetics than in the juvenile type. This may not actually be the case, however, because in the not too distant past a youngster with diabetes had very little likelihood of surviving to adulthood to produce children of his own. The person who did not get diabetes until middle age, however, probably had already had children and had passed on any tendencies to get the disease. Children of diabetic parents or grandparents are certainly at greater risk than the normal population, particularly if those offspring are overweight. The genetic link for juvenile diabetes may well exist at least in terms of the ability to acquire the disease if other conditions are right. There do seem to be loci (*B8* and *Dw3*) on the HLA region on chromosome 6 which are associated with risk of diabetes. On the other hand, no insulin-dependent diabetic has been found who has HLA-*Dw2*. These relationships are, however, purely statistical.

Why would insulin-dependent diabetes continue to be carried in the population at such high frequency (5%)? It is probably safe to assume that the insulin-dependent (juvenile) type could be a random event because left untreated, the disease is fatal before the reproductive years. The insulin-independent type, on the other hand, does not usually surface until after the prime child-bearing years. In addition this class of diabetics may be metabolically more efficient; they certainly are often overweight before the disease becomes manifest. During periods of time when food is scarce, there may be a selective advantage to being prediabetic. Short food supply was prevalent during much of man's evolutionary history, there could have been strong selective pressures in favor of diabetics. Even in modern times when food supplies are short, there are few reported cases of diabetes. Such was the case during World War II when food was unavailable to large segments of various European populations. When the food supplies stabilized then the frequency of diabetes in these populations returned to prewar levels. The metabolic efficiency and selective genetic pressures may account for the relatively high incidence of this disease in our society.

The diabetic suffers from an impairment of glucose uptake into tissues, excess glucose synthesis via gluconeogenesis and glycogenolysis, excess lipolysis, impaired lipogenesis, excess ketogenesis, and excess proteolysis. All of these impairments contribute to the large number of complications associated with the diabetic syndrome. It is often difficult, however, to correlate these complications with the type or severity of the disease. There is considerable deterioration of the peripheral vasculature which in itself has some severe consequences. For example, the destruction of capillaries in the retina of the eye (retinopathy) may result in blindness. Microvascular damage may cause kidney damage and ultimately renal failure, which is the second leading cause of death in diabetics. Once protein from the microvascular damage to the kidney is detected in the urine, the prognosis is poor. Dialysis or kidney transplants may prolong the ultimate consequences. When the destruction occurs in the extremities, hardening of the arteries also takes place further exacerbating the problem. Circulation becomes extremely impaired. Then, if there is an insult or trauma in this region (e.g., a blister or injury to a toe), a bacterial infection can gain ground to the point that gangrene may be the inevitable result. In this case, the diabetic will likely lose a toe, foot, or leg depending on the severity of the infection.

Vascular damage also makes a diabetic more prone to cardiovascular disease, the leading cause of death in diabetics. The pattern of vessel occlusion is, however, somewhat different than what is observed in a person with primary cardiovascular disease. In a diabetic the constriction of the vessels is far more likely to be peripheral than central. The danger is, of course, that a clot will form peripherally then migrate to a major artery in the heart or brain resulting in a heart attack or cerebrovascular accident.

Why would diabetics be more prone to cardiovascular disease than the general population? Non-insulin-dependent diabetics may have levels of circulating insulin higher than normal individuals. It is possible that the insulin itself is responsible for the secondary effect on the arteries. Some arterial damage may be immune in nature, and it has been suggested that repeated immunizations could cause the immune system to damage its own arteries. Repeated insulin injections might trigger a similar response. A viral infection could perhaps trigger the onset of both diabetes and vascular disease. The two syndromes could be casually related via abnormal serum lipid levels. Hyperlipidemia is frequently noted in diabetics. In insulin-dependent diabetics, lipoprotein lipase activity is low and clearance of serum triglycerides is therefore reduced. In insulin-independent diabetics triglyceride production may be increased. Serum cholesterol levels are less commonly elevated and sometimes the elevations may be in HDL cholesterol, which is thought to be a beneficial factor in the prevention of arterial damage. The best method for treating the lipid disorders of diabetes is good glycemic control.

Much of the time a diabetic may not be aware that he has sustained a peripheral injury. For that reason, a slight injury may get out of hand before it is noticed. This lack of detection arises because of another complication of diabetes, *peripheral neuropathy*. There is sufficient nerve damage to impair conduction velocity of signals along the nerve, and thus, signal transmission is limited. The neuropathy can ultimately lead to tissue damage because the lack of good nerve impulses may cause relatively poor coordination, tripping, and stubbing ones toes. Further, there may be little sense of pain and thus an unawareness of the damage. For this reason, diabetics are advised to make careful daily inspections of their feet and to always wear proper, good-fitting shoes and socks. The nerve damage may also be associated with loss of gastrointestinal tract function. Ultimately, passage of material through the tract is slowed, leading to a deterioration in GI function. Diabetics with neuropathy may benefit little from high fiber diets due to poor GI motility.

Most of the complications of diabetes can be attributed directly to the hyperglycemia associated with the disease. A number of pathways and processes are altered as the result of continued elevation of blood glucose. The known or conjectured effects of high blood glucose levels are detailed below.

One of the complications of diabetes is cataract formation, the opacity and swelling of the lens of the eye. Insulin is not required for glucose entry into the lens. The excess glucose can be converted to sorbitol by aldose reductase which also requires NADPH. Sorbitol cannot readily diffuse out of the lens so its accumulation results in osmotic swelling. The swelling results in an influx of sodium ions which exacerbates the problem. Ultimately, the lens fibers are disrupted resulting in cataracts. Drugs that inhibit aldose reductase have been successfully used to retard cataract formation in diabetic rats.

Another consequence of elevated blood glucose is glycosylation (enzymatic and nonenzymatic) of serum proteins. Nonenzymatic glycosylation of proteins occurs by means of Schiff base formation and an Amadori rearrangement to form a 1-amino-1-deoxyfructose. Other glycosylations are believed to be via analogous ketoamine linkages. Thus, the N-terminus and lysine residues are particularly suceptible to this reaction. The extent to which this process occurs depends on the concentration of blood glucose.

Glycosylated proteins are functionally different than nonglycosylated, native proteins. In the case of glycosylated hemoglobin, there is lowered oxygen affinity. There is also impaired binding of 2,3-diphosphoglycerate, which decreases oxygen release to the tissues. There may be as much as a 50% decline in these altered hemoglobins ability to deliver oxygen to the tissues. Another nonenzymatic glycosylation that may have considerable consequences for the diabetic is the addition of glucose to low density lipoproteins, which may contain from 1–10 moles of glucose per mole of protein. Glycosylation of these proteins impairs their ability to participate in the normal tissue turnover of cholesterol.

Enzymatic glycosylation can also be altered in the diabetic. In this process, lysine is converted to hydroxylysine, then a carbohydrate moiety is attached. In diabetics, lysine hydroxylase activity is increased and there may be an elevation of glucosyl- or galactosyl-transferase. This process is particularly important to the basement membrane of vessel walls. In diabetics this membrane thickens as a response to being glycosylated. The thickening undoubtedly reduces nutrient transfer to the tissues.

Micro- and macrovascular disease poses a serious risk to the diabetic. Some of the changes in serum proteins and the basement membrane may promote cardiovascular disease. Virchow's hypothesis that atherosclerosis is the body's response to arterial injury seems plausible in the case of the diabetic. The progress of the syndrome would be (1) endothelial injury, (2) platelet adherence, (3) platelet aggregation, (4) release of platelet substances that promote smooth muscle cell proliferation, (5) accumulation of extracellular matrix, (6) accumulation of lipids, and finally, (7) calcification. The injury might well result from an autoimmune attack on the glycosylated proteins that the body assumes to be foreign.

Neuropathy can also be the result of hyperglycemia. Nearly 80% of all diabetics have electrophysiological or morphological changes of the peripheral nerves. There may be several factors involved. Insulin is necessary for nearly all phases of the synthesis of complex lipids necessary to nerve function. Therefore, diabetes may impede the normal synthesis of nerve constituents. The second problem again relates to the accumulation of sorbitol via aldose reductase and fructose via sorbitol dehydrogenase. Accumulation of these polyols leads to fluid accumulation, increased pressure and nerve damage.

In retinopathy, regional ischemia due to poor oxygen release from hemoglobin is the central problem. Initially, there is a compensatory increase in the volume and number of vessels along with vessel dilation. A plasma skimming effect may occur. There are then formation of microaneurisms and vessel occlusion. Eventually, there is a breakdown of the blood–retinal barrier. In the early stages the problem is self-correctable by good glycemic control. Later, however, only surgery is useful. Renal pathology is very similar to the sequence of events for retinopathy.

B. TREATMENT MODALITIES

Diabetes is usually detected initially by screening for high glucose levels in urine or blood or when a patient complains of excessive thirst, hunger, and frequent urination.

To confirm the presence of the disease, an oral glucose tolerance test is administered. In this test a 50 or 75 g glucose (liquid) load is administered orally in a set time period. The test dose is given after a 12-hr fasting period. Blood glucose levels are then determined at fasting and 30 min, 1, 2, and 3 hr after glucose consumption. Values are compared to age matched controls. A typical glucose tolerance curve is shown in Fig. 12.1.

Since glucose tolerance deteriorates with age, it is important that adjustments be made in the curve for age of the patient. Other parameters affect the validity of the test as well. Since glucose tolerance is progressively impaired as the day progresses, it is important to administer the test in the early morning. There must be no other complicating factors such as fever, undue stress, or pregnancy. The patient also

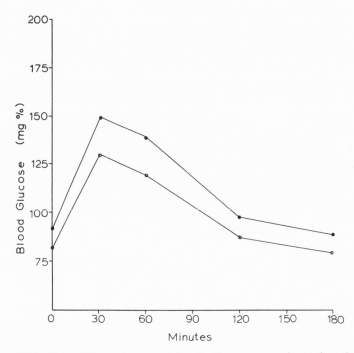

FIG. 12.1. Blood glucose determinations are made at time 0 after a 12 hr fast, then at 30, 60, 120, and 180 minutes after consuming a known quantity of a glucose solution. Curves indicate (○) typical 30- to 40-year old; (●) typical 40- to 80-year old.

must have consumed at least 150 g of carbohydrate for the three days previous to the 12-hr fast because carbohydrate consumption alters glucose tolerance. Even then, for certain diagnosis, a positive test requires either a follow-up glucose tolerance test or some independent diagnosis of diabetes.

Once the presence of the disease has been confirmed, a treatment modality must be selected. The present goal in treatment is to return blood glucose levels to "normal." If the victim is overweight, return to normal weight frequently results in the loss or amelioration of symptoms. Diet is the next line of defense. The usual diet for a diabetic contains a normal amount of protein (except in renal patients), reduced fat, with unsaturated fats comprising the bulk of the allowable fat, and about 50% of the calories as complex carbohydrates. Simple carbohydrates are to be avoided. Somewhat paradoxically, consumption of complex carbohydrates improves glucose tolerance. This may not be due to the carbohydrate per se but rather to the fact that such diets are frequently high in fiber content. Thus, the fiber itself, or some other agent in these diets, may be the actual factor that alters glucose tolerance.

Reducing stress may also make treatment easier. Individuals under stress secrete more glucocorticoids, which essentially antagonize the action of insulin. When stress is reduced, glucocorticoid secretion is diminished, thereby lowering the antagonism with insulin and improving treatment response.

If reduction of stress, weight loss, and diet modification are insufficient to promote return to normal blood glucose levels, then oral agents may be tried. Oral agents are not prescribed quite as frequently now as they once were because of the concern that there might be increased risk of cardiovascular abnormalities with the use of these drugs. Oral agents fall into two chemical categories: the sulfonylureas, of which tolbutamide is typical and the biguanide such as phenformin. These drugs often have side effects as the result of interactions with other agents. Further, they work only for insulin-independent diabetics.

Sometimes individuals who have been able to treat their diabetes with any of the above means become insulin dependent or they may fall into the category of insulin-dependent diabetics. If this is the case, there is presently no alternative to daily administration of insulin. Since insulin is a protein and therefore digested to its constituent amino acids in the G.I. tract, oral administration is not possible, and the insulin must be injected.

The frequency of the insulin shots required depends on several parameters. Too few injections could lead to wide swings in blood glucose levels and poor control of the disease. Too many injections increases the risk of infection at the injection site and the possibility of errors in the dosage. The sites of injection must be rotated to prevent two common but opposite problems around the site of injection: atrophy and hypertrophy. An individual taking several shots a day will have to use the same sites more frequently.

Part of the problem about frequency of injection is moderated by mixing insulins with different time courses of action. These may be mixtures of fast (regular or semilente), intermediate (globin, NPH, or lente) or slow acting (protamine zinc or ultralente) insulins. Another problem with insulins is that until recently commercial types were mostly from animals. Since these insulins are "foreign" proteins, it is possible to develop an allergic reaction to them. In terms of their antigenicity, insulin from beef or sheep are approximately equal and greater than pork insulin, which is greater than horse insulin. When an allergy develops to insulin from one species, it is sometimes possible to switch to insulin from a different species to resolve the problem. Newer techniques for isolating insulin from animal serum have resulted in purer preparations less prone to produce an allergy. An even more recent development should eliminate the problem of allergy entirely. Gene splicing is making it possible to make microorganisms produce large quantities of human insulin. Such insulin preparations should be reasonably free of antigenic activity.

Several alternatives are being developed to a continuous round of insulin shots. One that is presently being tested is the insulin pump. A permanent indwelling catheter is implanted in the abominal region and attached to a small external pump worn on the belt. The pump can be set to inject small doses of insulin at regular intervals and can be used to add extra insulin depending on the physiological state of the individuals. These pumps seem particularly promising for diabetics who have had difficulty maintaining good blood glucose control or who require multiple daily shots. More sophisticated models that monitor blood glucose and adjust the insulin dose accordingly may eventually become widely available.

The other alternative is still experimental and has yet to be shown to be feasible. It involves transplantation either of an intact pancreas or of functioning islets or β cells. Should such a treatment become routine, it would eliminate the need for external monitoring and insulin adjustment.

Diabetics may monitor the progress of their treatment several ways. First, there should be an abolition of gross symptoms such as excessive thirst, hunger, or urination and treatment should not cause faintness, mental confusion, or depression. Until recently, diabetics were advised to test their urine frequently for glucose using chemically treated test strips. A problem with this technique is that there may be a relatively poor correlation between blood glucose levels and the amount of glucose spilled from the kidneys into the urine. A preferred monitoring procedure is determination of blood glucose itself. This is accomplished by pricking the finger to get a drop of blood and using a test strip for the glucose determination. The usefulness of these techniques depends on the frequency with which they are performed. A diabetic may be out of glycemic control for a large percentage of the time without realizing it. A better indicator of overall control is determination of glycosylated hemoglobin. This is essentially a record of the control of blood glucose over the life-span of a red blood cell. It is not, however, a "home" procedure. Periodic glucose tolerance tests should also be used in conjunction with evaluation of treatment. Present evidence suggests that aggressive management of hyperglycemia vastly improves the prognosis for a diabetic and may result in a diminution of the side effects of the disease.

C. POSSIBLE CAUSES

There are several models for studying the causes, etiology, and outcomes of diabetes. One may, of course, attempt to study the disease in human volunteers. This approach poses several problems. First, it is unethical to induce diabetes in volunteers. It is also unethical to withhold beneficial treatment from individuals who have spontaneously contracted the disease. These limitations curtail the usefulness of human studies considerably. There are also a limited number of parameters that can be studied in large groups of human subjects under current guidelines for investigations using humans as experimental subjects.

There are several animal models that answer some of these objections. One might study an animal that develops diabetes spontaneously such as the Egyptian sand rat. Unfortunately, there are relatively few species of animals that have a high percentage of the population getting diabetes, and the ones who do are expensive and somewhat difficult to work with.

Chemically induced diabetes in common laboratory animals (rats) has also served as a model. Alloxan and streptozotocin are both diabetic agents said to destroy β cell function. These chemicals may also cause other damage, however, which could alter interpretation of results. Further, both undeniably cause a rise in blood glucose, but different mechanisms may be involved than are seen in spontaneous, "natural" diabetes. Low insulin levels may also be brought about by injecting anti-insulin serum, which binds normal insulin. Use of this antibody produces only a temporary diabetic state.

Another technique of some promise is the use of isolated organs or cells maintained in chemically defined media. In this way, hormone concentrations can be varied in a known manner and the changes observed in the absence of unknown, complicating factors. It is just these factors that occur in the whole animal though that may mediate various hormonal effects relevant to the disease. This model, too, then has its shortcomings. Together, all of the approaches (human, animal, and cell culture) may be expected to shed considerable light on the problem.

There are a number of potential causes of diabetes. It is likely that, in common with cancer or the common cold, the symptoms that arise and are termed diabetes could be in reality the result of several different syndromes. There may be a genetic component that determines whether external assaults will result in diabetes. Destruction of β cells, of course, would be expected to result in diabetes. This destruction could come about because of an autoimmune disease where the host attacks its own cells. The disease may come about as the result of a defect in synthesis and/or release of insulin. There could be several defects here. Normal proinsulin with the cleavage sites for C-peptide is shown in Fig. 12.2. C-peptide is a 30–35 amino acid peptide. A defective insulin may be produced in normal quantities or normal insulin may be produced in suboptimal quantities. A low quantity of insulin might result from impaired synthesis or from posttranslational problems. Since preproinsulin → proinsulin → insulin + C-peptide, an impairment of cleavage at either of these points would lower insulin levels. Insulin is packaged into β granules in preparation for fusion of granules with the cell membrane whereupon it is released into circulation. If there is a problem with the packaging or releasing mechanisms, then low insulin levels would result.

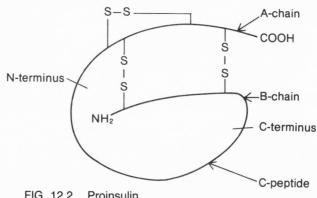

FIG. 12.2.   Proinsulin

Normal insulin in normal quantities may leave the β cell in a proper response to a secretion stimulus, but something may happen to it once it has left the β cell. An autoimmune phenomenon could cause host antibodies to attack the circulating insulin as foreign. Much of the circulating insulin is cleared by liver. If clearance is too rapid then low insulin levels would result in a diabetic syndrome. The half-life of proinsulin in the serum is about 20 min whereas the half-life of native insulin is about 5 min. There is no evidence for conversion of proinsulin to insulin in the serum.

The next level of defects resides at the level of cellular interaction with insulin. Insulin may be unable to bind properly with cellular receptors. There may be too few receptors, or antibodies to the receptors, or the receptors themselves may bind insulin satisfactorily but no subsequent event occurs. It is also possible that the insulin receptor interaction is functional and that a normal cellular "message" is sent but that the cell is unable to translate the message.

A further way to produce diabetes would be for the insulin to be synthesized, secreted, received, and translated normally but to have abnormal levels of counterregulatory hormones. For instance, insulin lowers blood glucose and glucagon raises it. If far more glucagon is produced than insulin, there will be a net rise in blood glucose and apparent diabetes. Other counterregulatory hormones such as glucocorticoids and epinephrine might be expected to cause a similar problem if produced in excess. Indeed, a number of stress-induced (or exacerbated) cases of diabetes have been described.

The study and treatment of disease in humans to date has primarily focused on returning blood glucose values to normal levels. Insulin, of course, has many functions in normal cellular processes. Besides regulating blood glucose levels, it also affects the uptake of certain amino acids and promotes activation of enzymes involved in fuel storage and inhibition of those associated with fuel degradation. Therefore, in the presence of insulin there is a net synthesis of glycogen and fat, and it aids in the storage of fat in the adipose tissue. It is widely assumed that a return of blood glucose to normal levels indicates a return of other insulin mediated processes to normal as well. Although this may be true in many cases, it is not necessarily true in all cases. Certainly, a great deal of further research will be needed before such a conclusion can be safely drawn.

D. SUMMARY

Diabetes is a common carbohydrate related disorder. In western societies about 5% of the population is afflicted. There are two prevalent types: insulin dependent and insulin independent. Diabetic complications include retinopathy, neuropathy, renal impairment, and increased risk of cardiovascular complications. The disease is characterized by high blood glucose levels and glucose in the urine with abnormal hunger, thirst, and urniation, and is diagnosed on the basis of abnormal glucose tolerance tests.

Treatment may include weight reduction, diet modification, and lowering of stress. Oral antidiabetagenic agents may be used in insulin-independent diabetes, but insulin administration is required for insulin-dependent diabetics.

Experimental models for study of this disease include human volunteers, animals that spontaneously develop diabetes, chemical induction of the disease, use of anti-insulin serum, or organ or cell culture in defined media. Although no single cause has been defined, diabetes may be the result of errors in the synthesis or release of insulin, destruction of normal insulin or inappropriate interaction of insulin with a cellular receptor, or improper translation of this interaction into a cellular event.

REVIEW QUESTIONS

1. What are the classifications of diabetes?
2. What are the treatment modalities?
3. What parameters affect oral glucose tolerance tests?
4. What are four complications of diabetes?

BIBLIOGRAPHY

DeFranzo, R.   1981.   Glucose tolerance and aging. Diabetes Care 4, 493–501.
Golberg, R.   1981.   Lipid disorders in diabetes. Diabetes Care 4, 561–572.
Goldstein, J., and Brown, M.   1977.   The low density lipoprotein pathway and its relation to atherosclerosis. Annu. Rev. Biochem. 46, 897–930.
Kolata, G.   1979.   Blood sugar and the complications of diabetes. Science 203, 1098–1099.
Reaven, G., and Steiner, G.   1981.   Proc. Conf. Diabetes and Atherosclerosis. Diabetes 30, Suppl. 2.

Salans, L., and Graham, B.   1982.   Task force on animals appropriate for studying
    diabetes mellitus and its complications. Diabetes *31*, Suppl. 1, Part 2.
Steiner, G.   1981.   Diabetes and atherosclerosis. Diabetes *30*, 1–7.
Sussman, D., and Metz, R.   1975.   Diabetes Mellitus, 4th Edition. American Diabetes
    Assoc. New York.
Unger, R.   1978.   Role of glucagon in the pathogenesis of diabetes: the status of the
    controversy. Metabolism *27*, 1691–1709.

13

Glycogen Storage Diseases

Excess glucose from the diet can be stored as glycogen. Lactate can also be converted to glycogen. In liver cells and, to a lesser extent, kidney cells, glycogen serves primarily as a repository of reserve glucose which can be put into the blood stream. In muscle and other tissues, glycogen serves as an endogenous supply of glucose for the cell and *cannot* contribute to blood glucose. One ordinarily thinks of liver and muscle as the primary sites of glycogen storage. Adipose tissue, however, has nearly as much glycogen as muscle when one considers adipose tissue on a fat-free basis.

In liver, glycogen levels under normal *ad libitum* feeding conditions are around 5% and can fall to less than 1% of the liver weight upon fasting. After fasting and refeeding a high carbohydrate diet, liver glycogen may become as high as 12% of the liver weight. The amount of muscle glycogen, on the other hand, is little affected by fasting per se, but is altered by exercise. Normally the level of muscle glycogen is about 2% of the muscle weight. Adipose tissue glycogen levels are similar to muscle levels if the weight of the fat is subtracted from the adipose tissue.

The pathways for synthesis and degradation of glycogen are discussed in Chapter 8. There are many glycogen storage diseases. This may not be surprising when one considers the multiple uses for glycogen depending on tissue location and the relative complexity of the regulation of the pathways for synthesis and degradation. The diseases are known by Roman numerals or in some cases by their eponyms. The types and the defects involved are shown in Table 13.1.

A. TYPE I—VON GIERKE'S DISEASE

This glycogen storage disease, a deficiency of glucose-6-phosphatase, has been recognized for quite a long time. It was first described in 1928 by von Gierke. This particular type of glycogen storage disease is by far the most prevalent, representing one-third of all the cases of this type of carbohydrate abnormality. Since the disease is caused by the absence of glucose-6-phosphatase, it affects liver and kidney, the two tissues containing this enzyme. The enzyme, which is found in the

TABLE 13.1.   The Glycogen Storage Diseases

Type	Name	Defect	Tissue affected
I	Von Gierke's disease	Glucose-6-phosphatase	Liver, kidney
II	Pompe's disease	Lysosomal glucosidase	All tissues
III	Cori's or Forbes disease	Debranching enzyme	Liver, muscle
IV	Andersen's disease	Branching enzyme	All tissues
V	McArdle's disease	Muscle phosphorylase	Skeletal muscle
VI		Liver phosphorylase	Liver
VII		Phosphofructokinase	Muscle
VIII		Low activity of liver phosphorylase due to low adenylate cyclase	Liver, brain
IX		Liver phosphorylase kinase	Liver
X		Cyclic AMP dependent phosphorylase kinase	Liver and muscle

microsomes, is responsible for the conversion of glucose 6-phosphate to glucose and phosphoric acid. It is the reverse of the hexokinase step except that no ATP is generated. This step is essential for conversion of glycogen to blood glucose.

The absence of glucose-6-phosphatase results in accumulation of glycogen in the liver and kidney, ultimately causing enlargement of these tissues. In this disease glucose cannot be formed from glycogen, and it also cannot be formed from amino acids or lactate since this enzymatic step is the last and crucial step in gluconeogenesis. Therefore, not only is glycogen metabolism impaired, but glucose production from other gluconeogenic precursors is also blocked.

The increase in glycogen concentration could be due to increased synthesis or to decreased breakdown of glycogen. Although the definitive evidence is still lacking, it is reasonable to suppose that the glycogen accumulation is due to an increased rate of synthesis. Recall that the inactive form of glycogen synthetase can become fairly active if there is a high level of glucose 6-phosphate which there is in this disease. Thus, glycogen can readily be synthesized by the glucose 6-phosphate dependent form of glycogen synthetase.

Growth is stunted in individuals with this defect. Since the liver cannot contribute glucose to the blood during hypoglycemia, the glucose 6-phosphate is converted instead to lactate to the point that lactic acidosis may occur. The low blood glucose levels cause the ratio of glucagon/insulin to rise, which in turn promotes adipose tissue lipolysis. Much of the fatty acid released is then reesterified in the liver. This causes a fatty liver in addition to the cellular hypertrophy caused by glycogen accumulation.

In spite of the severity of the disease, it is possible to survive if frequent small meals containing glucose are administered. The patient must avoid a high protein diet since gluconeogenesis is blocked.

B. TYPE II—POMPE'S DISEASE

Type II glcogen storage disease is due to a lack of the lysosomal enzyme $\alpha(1\rightarrow4, 1\rightarrow6)$-glucosidase and was first described in 1932. This enzyme is contained in the lysosome and hydrolyzes both $\alpha(1,4)$ and $\alpha(1,6)$ linkages with hydrolysis of the $\alpha(1,6)$ linkage proceeding at a slower rate. Since the enzyme can degrade both kinds of linkages, it is capable of completely hydrolyzing glycogen.

In early described cases of Pompe's disease, considerable attention was given to involvement of the heart muscle and, for a while, it was called *cardiomeglia glycogenica*. Now, however, it is known that there is widespread involvement of other tissues. There are three forms of the disorder: infantile, secondary, and adult. The infantile form is the most common and results in death by cardiorespiratory failure at a few months of age. There is extensive damage to muscle fibers and enlargement of the heart and liver with large accumulations of glycogen in the cytoplasm of cells. The response of glycogen metabolism to hormones is normal. The secondary form is not manifested until early childhood and progresses at a slower rate than the infantile form. Nevertheless, it is invariably fatal by 20 years of age. The adult form is much milder and usually not fatal although patients experience muscular weakness. Unlike the infantile form, there is little cytoplasmic glycogen accumulation in the adult form.

The disease is especially interesting from the standpoint of what we usually consider important in the normal synthesis and degradation of glycogen via the synthetase and phosphorylase systems. If the phosphorylase system is the primary route for glycogen degradation, one would not expect to find any severe debilitation due to the lack of the lysosomal enzyme.

Interpretation is complicated by data that suggest that at least part of the α-glucosidase is soluble rather than lysosomal. This does not rule out the possibility that victims of this disease may also have more fragile lysosomal membranes, which allow the enzyme to escape into the less favorable environment of the cytoplasm. Further, some adults have been shown to have an almost total lack of α-glucosidase without having any severe symptomology at all. It is clear that considerable work must be conducted to settle several important questions such as (1) is the α-glucosidase that is important in the disease actually sequestered in the lysosomes, and (2) what is the role of the enzyme in normal glycogen degradation?

C. TYPE III—CORI'S OR FORBES DISEASE

Type III glycogen storage disease is a lack of debranching enzyme. Although the disease is usually considered systemic, several studies have reported that some patients had a deficiency of debranching enzyme in liver, and normal enzyme in muscle or vice versa. It is not possible to decide at present whether debranching enzyme in liver and muscle is under the control of one gene with modifying factors present in a specific tissue or whether there are multiple enzymes which are tissue specific.

In this disease the glycogen molecules look like limit dextrins. Phosphorylase can remove all the terminal $\alpha(1,4)$ arms but a lack of debranching enzyme brings glycogen degradation to a halt at $\alpha(1,6)$ branch points. Debranching enzyme has in fact two activities: it is a transferase, removing maltotriose units to the 4 position of the non-reducing end of an acceptor chain and it is an amylo-1,6-glucosidase that attacks the exposed $\alpha(1,6)$ bond. Efforts to show that these two activities in reality reside in two separate proteins have so far been unsuccessful.

In patients with this syndrome, it is possible to deduce their recent nutritional pattern based on examination of their glycogen molecules. If the patients have recently been fed, the glycogen appears normal. If they are fasted, the glycogen resembles a limit dextrin. These patients do not respond normally to glucagon and epinephrine. Although there are some clinical symptoms associated with the disease (hepatomegaly, glycogen accumulation in the heart and other cells, and growth retardation) this disease need not be fatal. The usual treatment is frequent feeding and ingestion of a high protein diet.

D. TYPE IV—ANDERSEN'S DISEASE

Type IV glycogen storage disease, which is a defect in branching enzyme is, unlike Type III, usually fatal by the age of 2. Fortunately, Type IV is very rare. Glycogen formation is affected in all tissues. Because of the fewer number of branch points the glycogen molecules are said to resemble amylopectin and the disease has been called amylopectinosis.

Patients with Andersen's disease suffer considerable enlargement of the liver. The enlargement is due, however, to cirrhosis rather than to glycogen deposition per se. The cirrhosis may come about as the result of the attack on the abnormal glycogen by "foreign-body" immune type reactions. In this sense, Type IV could be called an autoimmune disease. It is somewhat odd that the failure to debranch glycogen is a mild disease whereas the failure to have a normal number of branches is fatal.

E. TYPE V—MCARDLE'S DISEASE

Type V glycogen storage disease involves a deficiency of muscle phosphorylase. The phosphorylase enzymes from muscle and liver are quite different indicating more than one gene is involved in coding for this enzyme activity. Therefore it is not surprising that the muscle enzyme can be affected whem the liver enzyme is not. In McArdle's disease, muscles are unable to use glycogen and must rely on fatty acids, amino acids, and blood glucose for their nutrient supplies. As a result patients are unable to perform heavy exercise. These patients are at a particular disadvantage during anaerobic exericse which relies on ATP generation from glycolysis because all the glycolysis must come from blood glucose. Because of the impaired glycolysis from glycogen, a rise in venous lactate is not observed in these patients during exercise. There is some accumulation of glycogen in muscle tissue.

The course of McArdle's disease is usually relatively mild with the treatment being avoidance of strenuous exercise. In evolutionary times, the diseases may have been removed from the population rather effectively by natural selection. Running from a fast-paced saber-toothed tiger probably effectively put an end to this defect in the population. Now, however, except for running to catch the bus, afflicted individuals can survive without undue difficulty. For this reason, it is likely that this disease may change in frequency from being relatively rare to being more frequent.

F. TYPE VI—HER'S DISEASE

The Type VI syndrome is similar to McArdle's disease except that it involves liver rather than muscle phosphorylase. Also similar is the fact that it too is relatively mild.

The disease can be detected by a glucagon response test. Naturally, patients with this defect do not show hyperglycemia in response to glucagon. Although the cyclic AMP–protein kinase–phosphorylase kinase part of the cascade is probably unimpaired, the lack of liver phosphorylase renders the degradation of glycogen in response to glucagon impossible.

Liver glycogen content increases in some but not all patients. There are also some hypoglycemia and reduced growth because the liver cannot contribute glucose to the blood from glycogen degradation. The disease is best treated by frequent feedings.

G. TYPE VII

Type VII glycogen storage disease is characterized by a lack of muscle phosphofructokinase, and would be expected to have more far-reaching consequences than just abnormal glycogen metabolism. The deficiency of this enzyme is rarely total; usually at least 5% of the activity is still present. Even so, during heavy exercise a build up of glucose 6-phosphate and fructose 6-phosphate occurs in the exercising muscle. Since muscles lack glucose-6-phosphatase, the intermediate metabolites become trapped in the pathway.

Some compensatory mechanisms develop in this disease. There is an increased oxygen carrying capacity of the blood brought about either by an increased hemoglobin concentration or by increased red cell production (or an increased half-life for the cells). There is a lack of one type of phosphofructokinase in the red cell itself. The increased oxygen capacity allows the muscle to function aerobically using fatty acids and amino acids exclusively for energy instead of relying on muscle glycogen.

H. TYPE VIII

Type VIII glycogen storage disease is a very rare disorder and its exact cause is unknown. This disease is characterized by anomalies in liver and brain glycogen storage and central nervous system damage. Although there is liver enlargement, glycogen deposition patterns are normal. In at least one case, there was low activity of phosphorylase and hypersecretion of catecholamines. The full activity of phosphorylase could be restored by injections of glucagon or epinephrine. It has been suggested that adenylate cyclase is deficient. If this is indeed the case, it would be expected that the regulation of a great many other enzymes would be altered as well. Further, in light of the demonstration that much of the action of epinephrine occurs via α receptors that are not linked to adenylate cyclase, it is difficult to rationalize a deficiency of adenylate cyclase.

I. TYPE IX

Type IX glycogen storage disease is marked by a deficiency of liver phosphorylase kinase. Thus, the normal regulation of glycogen degradation is impaired. There appears to be two methods of inheritance of this disease: autosomal recessive and X-linked recessive.

The disease is mild and is usually associated with asymptomatic hepatomegaly. Biochemical abnormalities, such as acidosis or hypoglycemia, are rare. There may even be some adaptation as the patient ages because the liver enlargement disappears. Growth retardation has been observed. A high protein diet is the recommended "cure."

J. TYPE X

There has been only one case reported (Tarui *et al.* 1969) of Type X glycogen storage disease. The disease appeared to be due to a deficiency of cyclic AMP dependent protein kinase. Such a deficiency, of course, would be expected to alter all the systems sensitive to this enzyme as well as the enzymes of the glycogen system. However, there are other protein kinases that are cyclic AMP independent which may partially compensate for this defect. In the one known case, the patient did not respond to glucagon and there was some liver enlargement. Otherwise, there were no overt symptoms.

K. SUMMARY

Glycogen synthesis and degradation involve a number of enzymatic steps and thus a number of defects in glycogen metabolism are theoretically possible. Ten have been identified so far. The most common type of glycogen storage disease is Type I, or von Gierke's disease, which is a lack of glucose-6-phosphatase. The other types range in frequency from relatively rare to extremely rare. These disease states may be the result of an absolute lack of enzyme, a deficient quantity of enzyme, or an adequate quantity of defective enzyme. The same symptomology may result regardless of the mechanism. The various diseases range from asymptomatic to fatal and may exhibit varying degrees of severity in the nonfatal cases even when the same lesion is involved. Different tissues may be affected or the disease may be generalized depending on whether the enzyme in question is the product of one gene locus or several.

REVIEW QUESTIONS

1. Which is the most common glycogen storage disease?
2. Why is phosphorylase deficiency tissue specific?
3. Which diseases are involved with glycogen branches? Which are fatal and which are mild?
4. What systems should be affected by Type VIII and X.

BIBLIOGRAPHY

Berdanier, C.   1976.   Genetic errors in carbohydrate metabolism. *In* Carbohydrate Metabolism. C. Berdanier (Editor) J. Wiley & Sons, New York.
Brown, D., and Brown, B.   1975.   Some inborn errors of carbohydrate metabolism. *In* Biochemistry of Carbohydrates. W. Whelan (Editor). Butterworths, London.
Hug, G.   1976.   Glycogen storage diseases. Birth Defects *12*, 145–175.

Huijing, F.   1975.   Glycogen metabolism and glycogen storage diseases. Physiol. Rev.
    55, 609–658.
McGilvery, R., and Goldstein, G.   1979.   Biochemistry. W. B. Saunders, Philadelphia,
    Pennsylvania.
Tarui, S., Kono, N., Nasu, T., and Nishikawa, M.   1969.   Enzymatic basis for the coex-
    istence of myopathy and hemolytic disease in inherited phosphofructokinase defi-
    ciency. Biochem. Biophys. Res. Commun. *34*, 77–83.

14

Lactose and Galactose Errors

A. LACTOSE INTOLERANCE

Lactose is the primary carbohydrate in most mammalian milk. The most notable exception is the sea lion (and some other marine mammals) whose milk contains no detectable carbohydrate. Most young mammals depend on milk as their predominant source of nutrients. Consumption of milk or milk based products may continue through adulthood in the case of humans and animals consuming commercial rations. School lunch programs in the United States and world feeding projects for the nutritionally inadequate have stressed the incorporation of milk in the dietary regimens. Powdered milk constitutes a major source of food being sent to underdeveloped countries.

In spite of the best of intentions of such programs, milk consumption may cause much of the world's population varying degrees of discomfort because the lactose in milk is poorly tolerated by many people. Symptoms may range from flatulence to mild G.I. tract discomfort to severe osmotic diarrhea. Disorders of lactose metabolism are unrelated to allergies to milk protein. The two maladies could, however, conceivably occur in the same individual.

There are several errors of lactose metabolism which may be separately defined (Table 14.1). Listed first is *congenital lactase deficiency*. This is caused by a lack of lactase in the intestinal mucosa of the GI tract and results in chronic acid diarrhea. Fortunately, this diease is very rare. *Lactose malabsorption* is detected using a glucose tolerance test. Since lactose is broken down into glucose and galactose by lactase, one should see a rise in blood glucose upon consumption of lactose if a normal amount of lactase is present in the GI tract. A flat glucose tolerance curve indicates malabsorption. *Primary lactase deficiency* (hypolactasia) is actually the normal condition of much of the world's human population and most adult mammals. The low level of lactase is consistent with the pattern one sees in lactase activity as a function of age; as age increases GI lactase acivity decreases. *Secondary lactase deficiency* is also a deficiency of lactase, but in this case it is the result of intestinal injury or a secondary result of another disease condition. *Lactose intolerance* is a general term to describe the discomfort symptoms that arise from the consumption of lactose.

TABLE 14.1.   Disorders of Lactose Metabolism

Error	Description	Symptoms
Congenital lactase deficiency	Lack of mucosal cell lactase, occurs neonatally	Chronic acid diarrhea
Lactose malabsorption	Detected by a flat glucose tolerance curve	Mild to severe
Primary lactase deficiency	Low intestinal lactase seen in older children and adults	Mild to severe
Secondary lactase deficiency	Low intestinal lactase as the result of injury or disease	Mild to severe
Lactose intolerance	General term used to describe discomfort symptoms arising from the consumption of lactose	

Problems with the metabolism of lactose are the result of an inappropriate amount of lactase, a β-galactosidase that cleaves lactose into equimolar amounts of glucose and galactose. Human small intestine contains three species of β-galactosidase: a neutral one (pH optimum of 6.0), a hetero-β-galactosidase inactive against lactose, and an acid one (pH optimum of 4.0). The neutral enzyme accounts for most of the lactose cleavage. It is found in highest activity in the brush border of the jejunum. The hetero-β-galactosidase is a cytoplasmic enzyme found in the intestinal epithelial cells. The acid enzyme is found in the lysosomes and may be involved in mucopolysaccharide and glycopeptide degradation. Neither of these enzymes contributes significantly to the metabolism of lactose.

All young mammals have higher lactase activity than older animals. Since milk is the primary nutrient source for the infant, it would be expected that the lactase activity of these animals should be high at birth in order to take advantage of the lactose contained in milk. Such is indeed the case. Lactase is not needed during prenatal life since lactose is not a nutrient source *in utero*. It is not surprising that lactase is one of the last enzymes to develop in the fetus. Lactase activity peaks shortly after birth then begins to steadily decline into adulthood (Fig. 14.1).

There appears to be a genetic linkage to lactose intolerance. Non-Caucasians are more susceptible than Caucasians. It has been estimated that 70% of the world population (adult) is lactose intolerant. Page *et al.* (1975) have examined the onset of intolerance in several populations and have found that 50% of Peruvians (mestizo) are intolerant by age three and 50% of the U.S. Black population is afflicted by age 13. Less than 20% of the U.S. white population becomes intolerant of lactose at any age. The degree of discomfort from a given quantity of lactose varies considerably with the individual. There may be little

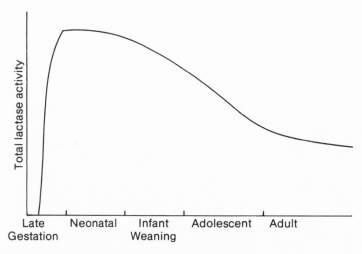

FIG. 14.1.   Lactase activity as a function of age.

discomfort from drinking an 8 oz. glass of milk in one person and severe consequences for such an indescretion in another.

Lactose intolerance is determined using a lactose tolerance test, which is very similar to the glucose tolerance test. In practice, a test load of lactose (50 g for adults and 2 g/kg for children) is administered after an overnight fast. Blood glucose values are determined at zero time and 15, 30, 60, 90, and 120 min after the test dose. This test may be subject to several errors. Some individuals peak very early, so it is important to take early (15 min) readings to avoid false positives. Diabetics may also give anomalous results. Since diabetics have exaggerated glucose responses, they may in fact be lactose intolerant and still show a normal glucose curve, thus giving false negatives.

Biopsy of the intestine to actually determine lactase activity is the most reliable means of detection. This is seldom used because of the obvious surgical risks. Usually it is much easier to remove the offending foods from the diet and to assume a deficiency of lactase when the lactose tolerance curve is abnormal.

Considerable attention has been given to the possibility of delaying, preventing, or reversing the onset of lactose intolerance. It has been suggested that continued consumption of milk and its products after weaning might delay or prevent the onset of lactose intolerance. Repeated studies have shown, however, that continued lactose consumption does not prevent the decrease in lactase activity. Further, cessation of lactose ingestion in normal individuals does not reduce lactase levels. If one is genetically predisposed to have this syndrome then the lactose content of the diet does not alter its course. If one is not genetically predisposed to develop this syndrome, the same is true. A number of claims have been made, however, that continued lactose ingestion increases lactose tolerance and lactase activity. In studies by Ekstrom and his co-workers (1975,1976), it was found that lactose consumption did not alter the lactase activity of the gut itself. It did, however, increase the lactase activity of the gut contents. Therefore, the "adaptation" effect that is sometimes seen is probably due to a change in the gut microflora population rather to a change in the quantity of intestinal lactase.

Efforts have been made to treat milk products in such a way as to make them "safe" for lactose intolerant individuals. These have included treating milk with lactase isolated from microorganisms. Consumption of this product by lactose intolerant individuals led to near normal tolerance curves. One important consideration in choosing methods to lower the lactose content of milk is the effect that such measures have on the taste and sensory qualities of the milk. Cheese products do not pose a significant problem because the lactose is essentially removed with the whey during the cheese making process. Yogurt and other fermented dairy products may also be tolerated by many lactose intolerant individuals. Although there is still some lactose in these products, fermentation lowers the lactose content. Dairy products represent a good source of many nutrients and are relatively easy to distribute worldwide. The high percentage of the world population having lactose intolerance, however, necessitates the modification of these products in such a way as to circumvent the genetic defect to prevent the suffering caused by lactose ingestion.

B. GALACTOSEMIA

There are two defects associated with the metabolism of galactose. One results from a lack of the ability to phosphorylate galactose and the other arises from the loss of ability to transfer the phosphorylated derivative.

When there is a deficiency of the *galactokinase* (a lack of the ability to phosphorylate galactose), the most common symptom is cateracts on the lens of the eye. This occurs because galactose accumulates and can be reduced by a nonspecific NADPH-linked aldose reductase to form galactitol (Fig. 14.2). The only route for disposal of this undesirable compound is via the urine. Since there is considerable aldose reductase in the lens of the eye, there is a buildup of galactitol in this tissue which results in osmotic swelling and ultimately in disruption of the lens fibers.

The consequences of the second defect, a deficiency of the *galactose-1-phosphate uridyltransferase,* are far more severe. This deficiency not only causes cataracts but liver, kidney, and organic brain damage as well. Fortunately, it is relatively easy to test for this disease. Red blood cells are assayed for the presence of the transferase. Indication that the activity of the transferase is low or absent requires

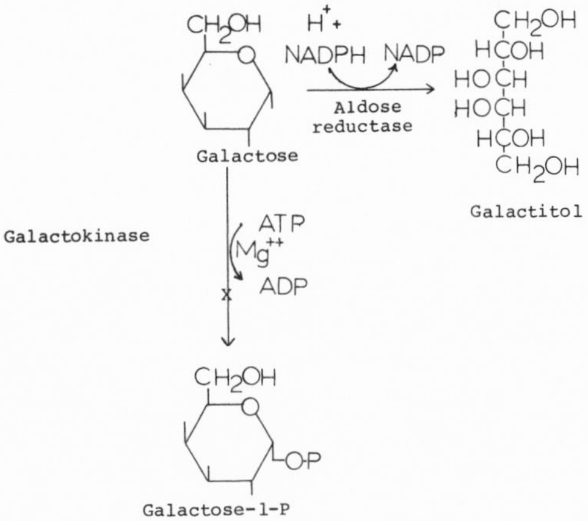

FIG. 14.2. Formation of galactitol from galactose in the absence of galactose kinase.

that the affected individual completely avoids any food containing galactose. Usually galactose 1-phosphate synthesis is unimpaired in these individuals.

A transferase deficiency is caused by an autosomal recessive defect. Therefore, one would expect to see a simple Mendelain inheritance pattern in a family of four children whose parents carry the defect: one galactosemic, two heterozygotes, and one normal. In the United States, it has been estimated that the incidence of this disease is rather high (1%) and that one in 35,000 children are symptomatic. Since there appears to be no selective advantage to the syndrome, it is not clear why it persists at such a high level in the population. There are some variants of the simple defect as well.

The toxic agent in transferase deficiency galactosemia is galactose 1-phosphate, which builds up because it cannot be converted ultimately to glucose after being transferred to UDP (Fig. 14.3). That galactose 1-phosphate is the culprit in the symptomology is inferred rather than actually tested by comparing the symptoms of galactokinase deficiency with those of transferase deficiency. When galactose 1-phosphate builds up, three reactions become blocked (Fig. 14.4). The transfer of glucose 1-phosphate to form UDPG for glycogen synthesis is blocked causing disturbances in glycogen metabolism. The mutase reversibly changing glucose 1-phosphate to glucose 6-phosphate is also inhibited. Finally, glucose-6-phosphate dehydrogenase, which forms 6-phosphogluconate as the first step in the hexose monophosphate shunt, is inhibited. This defect limits NADPH production, which is necessary for such synthetic processes as cholesterol and fatty acid syntheses. Therefore, it can be seen that a defect in the transferase has more far-reaching consequences than the inability to form galactose 1-phosphate due to a loss of the kinase. If the kinase is missing, normal body function is not greatly impaired as galactose is not used at all, but if it

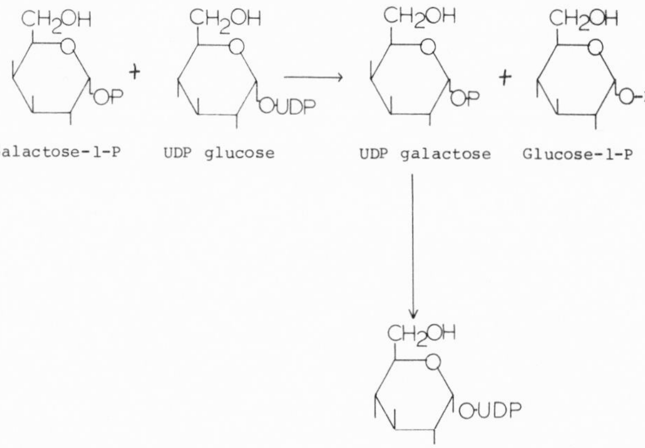

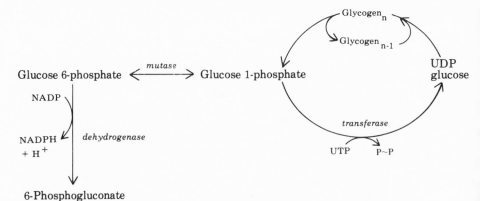

FIG. 14.3.   The galactose-1-phosphate uridyltransferase reaction.

FIG. 14.4.   Blocks in normal metabolic pathways caused by a buildup of galactose 1-phosphate.

is partially used (converted to galactose 1-phosphate) and the transferase is absent, the body is unable to cope with the intermediate
product.

C. SUMMARY

Lactose intolerance is caused by a low level of lactase activity in the
brush border of the small intestine due either to a congenital defect or
secondary, to an injury or disease of the GI tract. Symptoms may range
from mild to severe, and the syndrome is usually detected by a lactose
tolerance curve. The usual treatment is avoidance of foods containing

lactose. There is a natural decline in lactase activity in mammals with aging which is unaffected by the presence or absence of lactase in the diet. There may be some apparent "adaptation" to dietary lactose because of a change in the gut microflora.

There are two defects associated with galactose metabolism. Both are referred to as galactosemia. A galactokinase deficiency is a relatively mild syndrome producing cateracts of the eye. The more severe condition is the result of a deficiency of galactose-1-phosphate uridyltransferase. Not only is there damage to the eye but there is also liver, kidney, and brain dysfunction as well. The trait is carried in the population at a rather high rate (1%), but the reason for this is not apparent. The treatment for these defects is avoidance of galactose containing foods.

REVIEW QUESTIONS

1. What are the diseases associated with lactose intolerance?
2. What enzymes are involved with lactose digestion?
3. Why do the two defects in galactose metabolism produce symptoms with such disparate severities?

BIBLIOGRAPHY

Ekstrom, K., Benevenga, N., and Grummer, R.   1975.   Effects of diets containing dried whey on the lactase activity of the small intestinal mucosa and the contents of the small intestine and cecum of the pig. J. Nutr. *105,* 851–860.

Ekstrom, K., Grummer, R., and Benevenga, N.   1976.   Effects of diets containing dried whey on the lactase activity of the intestine and cecum of hampshire and chester white pigs. J. Anim. Sci. *42,* 106–114.

Gray, S.   1975. Oligosaccharides of the small intestinal brush border. *In* Physiological Effects of Food Carbohydrates. ACS Symp. Ser. 15. Am. Chem. Soc., Washington, D.C.

Greene, H.   1979.   Carbohydrate absorption. *In* Developmental Nutrition. K. Oliver, B. Cox, T. Johnson, and W. Moore (Editors). Ross Laboratories, Columbus, Ohio.

Johnson, T., Moore, W., and Jeffries, J.   1978.   Children Are Different, 2nd Edition. Ross Laboratories, Columbus, Ohio.

Kretchmer, N.   1972.   Lactose and lactase. Sci. Am. *227,* 70–78.

Paige, D., Bayless, T., Haung, S.-S., and Wexler, R.   1975.   Lactose intolerance and lactose hydrolyzed milk. *In* Physiological Effects of Food Carbohydrates. A. Jeanes and J. Hodge (Editors). ACS Symp. Ser. 15. Am. Chem. Soc., Washington, D.C.

Pike, R., and Brown, M.   1975.   Nutrition: An Integrated Approach, 2nd Edition J. Wiley & Sons, New York.

Winick, M.   1972.   Nutrition and Development. J. Wiley & Sons, New York.

15

Other Errors of Carbohydrate Metabolism

A. FRUCTOSE INTOLERANCE

Fructose is found in fruit and honey and constitutes 50% of sucrose and invert sugar. Approximately 40% of the wet weight of honey is fructose, and fruits and berries contain about 5% fructose. This sugar has become increasingly popular as a sweetener which is due in part to economical commercial methods for its production. There is widespread belief, fueled by dubious advertising, that fructose has less calories than sucrose. In point of fact all carbohydrates have about 4 cal/g. Under some, but not all, conditions fructose may be perceived to be sweeter. A calorie saving would result if less fructose could be used to attain a given degree of sweetness. Whether fructose is truly sweeter than sucrose depends on its physical state. The greatest degree of sweetness from fructose is perceived when the sugar is in a cold, dilute solution at neutral or slightly acidic pH.

Most commercial fructose, which is used as a tabletop sweetner or in processed foods, is prepared from cornstarch. The increasingly wide use of fructose has precipitated concern about its overall effect on health and its impact on the people who are genetically incapable of dealing with it. At one time fructose was popularized as a sweetner acceptable in diets for diabetics. Since fructose is almost entirely filtered out by the liver after it enters from the digestive tract and since insulin is not required for its entry into cells, it was reasoned that fructose would be a good substitute for glucose. Unfortunately, fructose is readily converted to glucose and hyperglycemia can easily occur in the diabetic when fructose is ingested. Metabolism of fructose may also result in a sufficient increase in serum lactate to contribute to acidosis.

The use of fructose in i.v. fluids and in parenteral regimens is dangerous. In humans there is so much lactate produced that blood pH falls when fructose is substituted for glucose in these fluids. Uric acid concentration rises as the result of high demand on the liver ATP pool (Fig. 15.1). In effect more AMP is produced leading to the degradation of adenine nucleotides to uric acid. There is, of course, a concomitant loss of inorganic phosphate which further disrupts the cellular ion

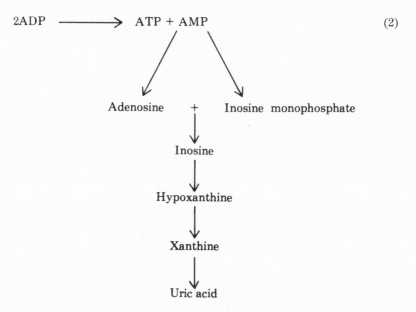

$$\text{Fructose} + \text{ATP} \longrightarrow \text{Fructose 1-phosphate} + \text{ADP.} \qquad (1)$$

$$2\text{ADP} \longrightarrow \text{ATP} + \text{AMP} \qquad (2)$$

Adenosine   +   Inosine monophosphate

Inosine

Hypoxanthine

Xanthine

Uric acid

FIG. 15.1.   The production of uric acid as the result of a fructose load.

balance. Even low rates of fructose infusion (0.5 g/kg body weight/hr) cause problems severe enough to cause liver failure and shock. The consequences are even more severe for diabetics. Because of all of these adverse side effects, fructose should not be used parenterally or intravenously.

Ordinarily, fructose is removed from the portal circulation by the liver. Very little free fructose ever escapes into general circulation. The liver removes fructose by phosphorylating it with ATP. The bulk of this phosphorylation is catalyzed by *fructokinase,* which produces fructose 1-phosphate. Some (a far lesser amount) of the fructose can be phosphorylated by hexokinase to produce fructose 6-phosphate, which can then proceed directly through glycolysis or be converted to glucose 6-phosphate for gluconeogenesis or glycogen synthesis. When fructose 1-phosphate is formed, it is first split into dihydroxyacetone phosphate (DHAP) and D-glyceraldehyde by *aldolase.* This is the same aldolase which cleaves fructose 1,6-bisphosphate. There are then two pathways available to enable the glyceraldehyde to enter glycolysis (Fig. 15.2). The triosekinase path is believed to be quantitatively more important.

Individuals with errors in fructose metabolism may have defects at

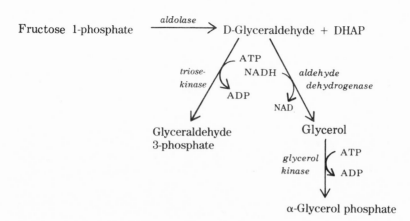

FIG. 15.2.   Metabolism of fructose-1-phosphate.

several steps. A lack of *fructokinase* leads to *fructosuria*. This is a relatively benign condition inherited as an autosomal recessive defect whose principal symptom is excretion of fructose in the urine. It is usually detected by using a total reducing sugar assay during screening for diabetes. The danger, of course, is that the individual would be mistakenly labeled as a diabetic. Urine tests specific for glucose and glucose tolerance tests would be necessary for confirmation of diabetes.

Fructose intolerance, on the other hand, is a far more serious disorder than fructosuria. Eating fructose containing foods results in vomiting, hypoglycemia, and ultimately in an enlarged liver and jaundice in individuals with this disease. This syndrome is due to a defect in the *aldolase* that cleaves fructose 1-phosphate. There are several isozymes of this enzyme with differing affinities for fructose 1,6-bisphosphate and fructose 1-phosphate. Type B, which is found in liver, has approximately equal affinities for both compounds. Fructose intolerance is not ordinarily detected until after weaning when fruits and sugar (sucrose) are introduced into the infant's diet. If the intolerance remains undetected, cirrhosis of the liver, mental retardation, and even death can be the result.

A further error is occasionally observed which is not restricted to fructose metabolism alone. This is a deficiency of *fructose 1,6-bisphosphatase*. Such a lack impairs not only the utilization of fructose for glucose synthesis but also gluconeogenesis from lactate or pyruvate. Since gluconeogenesis is impaired, one sees a fasting hypoglycemia in this condition. Lactate builds up and spills into the serum causing metabolic acidosis. The first case of this deficiency was reported in 1970, and a few other cases have subsequently been discovered. An insufficient number of cases have been studied to determine the optimum treatment. This deficiency must be presently regarded as potentially fatal.

B. MUCOPOLYSACCHARIDE DISORDERS

Study of genetic disorders of mucopolysaccharide metabolism is complicated because the pathways of metabolism of mucopolysaccharides are less well characterized than many other reactions of carbohydrate metabolism. Since most of the mucopolysaccharides are concentrated in connective tissue, it has been difficult to find a model organ for study since there is none that is composed primarily of connective tissue. The development of tissue cultures of fibroblasts has greatly aided the study of mucopolysaccharidoses because these cultured cells are predominately responsible for producing the mucopolysaccharides found in connective tissue.

Near the end of World War I, Hunter described a severely disfiguring syndrome. A few years later more cases were noted which showed not only the disfigurement but also corneal clouding and mental retardation. The disease came to be known as Hurler's syndrome or *gargoylism* and was believed to be a disorder of lipid metabolism. Not until the 1950s was it discovered that the disorder was really an error of mucopolysaccharide metabolism. The material that accumulated, causing the ridged skin, coarse features, clawed hands, hepatosplenomegaly, dwarf stature, corneal opacity, brain damage, and early death, was heparin sulfate. The material was found to accumulate in the lysosomes even though the rates of synthesis and excretion of mucopolysaccharides were normal. Using fibroblasts from normal and Hurler's syndrome patients, it was concluded that the defect was due to a lack of α-L-iduronidase. With this defect, one is unable to hydrolyze iduronic acid residues from heparin or dermatin chains.

There are in reality a number of variants of Hurler's syndrome (MPSIH). One of the milder forms is Hunter's syndrome (MPSII). It is different from the other mucopolysacchridoses in that it is an X-linked recessive genetic disease. In this disease there is also an accumulation of dermatin and heparin sulfate but the symptoms are not so severe, and there is rarely any eye damage. Although evidence is not conclusive, this disease is probably the result of a 2-sulfo-L-iduronate sulfatase deficiency.

Scheie syndrome, MPSIS, is also a variant of Hurler's disease. Patients inhibit corneal clouding, aortic valve damage, and deformity. In contrast to those afflicted with Hurler's disease, however, these patients not only have a normal life-span but also normal or superior intelligence instead of brain damage. Scheie disease is also a lack of α-L-iduronidase. Since the two diseases are not alike, however, there must be some information lacking about this enzyme and its regulation.

Sanfilippo syndrome (MPS IIIA and IIIB) is also one of the mucopolysaccharidoses. Patients with this defect escape most of the skeletal deformities but suffer instead impairments of the central nervous system. They excrete large amounts of heparin sulfate, which has a high

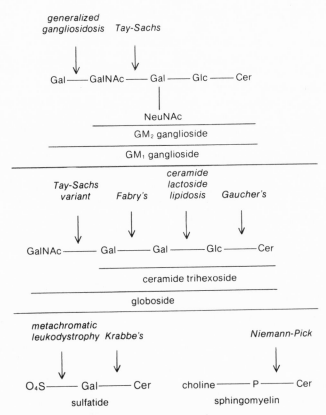

FIG. 15.3.   Defects in some lipid storage diseases.
Reprinted with permission from McGilvery and Goldstein (1979).

content of N-sulfo groups. The Type A form of the disease is presently considered to be a lack of N-sulfo-D-glucosamine sulfatase. The Type B form is probably due to a deficiency of α-N-acetylglucosaminidase.

Other types of mucopolysaccharidoses have been described, including Morguio syndrome and Maroteaux–Lamy syndrome. The symptoms and excretion products are known, but the sites of the defects have not yet been determined.

C. LIPID STORAGE DISEASES

Usually lipid storage diseases are considered to be defects of lipid metabolism. In fact, they are errors in the lysosomal degradation of the carbohydrate portion of the glycolipids (Fig. 15.3).

One of the most widely recognized of these syndromes is *Tay–Sachs disease,* which has an especially high incidence among the Ashkenazic

Jewish population. The disease leads to blindness and progressive central nervous system deterioration. This disorder is the result of a defect in the enzyme *hexosaminidase* which cleaves *N*-acetylgalactosamine from gangliosides. Partially degraded ganglioside builds up causing the difficulty. There are several variants of this disease depending on the position of the *N*-acetylgalactosamine attacked.

Another defect occurring with some frequency in Jewish populations is the autosomal recessive disorder, *Gaucher's disease*. In this disease glucosylceramide builds up, especially in the spleen and liver. The ability to hydrolyze the bond between the glucose and ceramide is impaired and, because of the defective *glucocerebrosidase,* abnormal gangliosides and globosides accumulate.

In *Fabry's disease,* there is an accumulation of galactosylgalactosylglucosylceramide due to a defect in α-*galactosidase*. This disease, which causes kidney or cardiac failure resulting in death, is relatively rare.

Krabbe's disease is a failure to split the galactose–ceramide bond of sulfatides. Like all of the other lipid storage diseases, the error is in a lysosomal enzyme. Lysosomes from such patients are deficient in the particular enzymes and also abnormal in structure. Sometimes these syndromes are called lysosomal storage diseases rather than lipid storage diseases. To be technically correct, it should be emphasized that it is usually the metabolism of the carbohydrate portions of these glycolipids which is in error.

D. SUMMARY

Fructose is gaining popularity as a sweetner and increasing interest has been generated in the consequences of its metabolism. Fructose cannot be used in i.v. or parenteral preparations because it causes severe lactic acidosis and uric acid production. Dietary fructose is very effectively sequestered by the liver through phosphorylation, primarily to fructose 1-phosphate. Several genetic defects in fructose metabolism may occur: fructosuria due to a lack of fructokinase, and fructose intolerance because of insufficient aldolase. The first condition is benign whereas the second is severe.

The mucopolysaccharide disorders have been more difficult to characterize biochemically because their metabolic pathways are less well defined. Hurler's syndrome is a result of a deficiency of L-iduronase. Although there is some doubt, it is believed that 2-sulfo-L-iduronate sulfatase deficiency causes Hunter's syndrome.

There are a number of lipid storage diseases that are due in reality to defects in the addition and subtraction of carbohydrate portions of the glycolipid. The accumulation of various abnormal glycolipids in tissues has an especially deleterious effect on the central nervous system.

REVIEW QUESTIONS

1. What are the consequences of using fructose in I.V. or parenteral preparations?
2. Why are lipid storage disease misnamed? Give examples.
3. What are the respective defects in fructosuria and fructose intolerance?
4. What enzyme(s) are defective in Hurler's disease and Scheie syndrome? Why are the symptoms different?

BIBLIOGRAPHY

Brady, R. 1973. Hereditary fat-metabolism diseases. Sci. Am. *229,* 88–97.

Brown, D., and Brown, B. 1975. Some inborn errors of carbohydrate metabolism. *In* Biochemistry of Carbohydrates. W. Whelan (Editor). Butterworths, London.

Cherrington, A. 1981. Gluconeogensis: its regulation by insulin and glucagon. *In* Handbook of Diabetes Mellitus, Vol. 3. M. Brownlee (Editor). Garland STPM Press, New York.

McGilvery, R., and Goldstein, G. 1979. Biochemistry. W. B. Saunders, Philadelphia, Pennsylvania.

Palm, J. 1975. Benefits of dietary fructose in alleviating the human stress response. *In* Physiological Effect of Food Carbohydrates. A. Jeanes and J. Hodge (Editors). ACS Symp. Ser. 15 Am. Chem. Soc., Washington D.C.

Stanbury, J., Wyngaarden, J., and Fredrickson, D. 1978. Metabolic Basis of Inherited Disease. J. Wiley & Sons, New York.

van den Berghe, G. 1978. Metabolic effects of fructose in the liver. Curr. Topics Cell. Regul. *13,* 97–137.

16

Sucrose Metabolism and Disease

A. SUCROSE AND THE MODERN WESTERN DIET

Sugar cane was first cultivated in India around 300 BC. Use of sugar spread westward only gradually, and it was not until the Middle Ages that sucrose became well known in Europe. Because it was still very expensive at that time, the use of sucrose was restricted to the very wealthy or as a sweetner to cover the bitter taste of medicines. Besides discovering the Americas in 1492, Columbus brought sugar cane to the Caribbean. Ultimately, this led to a flourishing sugar industry, which brought the use of sugar within the reach of the less wealthy of Europe. Still further substantial reductions in cost resulted from the development of sugar beet technology in the late nineteenth century leading to the use of sugar as a cheap, abundant source of calories in the Western diet. Until 1925 there was a continued increase in sucrose consumption. Since then the level of consumption in Western societies has remained stable at approximately 18% of the total calories. The proportion of complex carbohydrates in the diet has declined during the period of increased sucrose consumption.

A number of disease states have been linked with sucrose consumption. Dental caries, diabetes, obesity, and heart disease are chief among these. Among the more fanatical food faddists, sucrose has also been suggested to cause hyperactivity in children and criminal behavior among adults, giving substance to the phrase "I'll kill for a piece of candy." Most of the evidence linking sucrose to caries, diabetes, obesity, and heart disease has been epidemiological.

With regard to the etilogy of heart disease, John Yudkin gave considerable impetus to sucrose consumption as a risk factor. In an article in *The Lancet* Yudkin (1963) listed a series of propositions paraphrased as follows: (1) any species is genetically suited to a particular diet; (2) animals will select those foods that meet their dietary requirements; (3) man is suited to a high protein, moderate fat, low carbohydrate diet; (4) palatibility is not identical with nutritional worth; (5) technology has separated nutritional worth and palatibility and; (6) the separation leads to over consumption of calories and metabolic disruptions which contribute to the development of the "modern ills" of man. Yudkin suggested that, since sucrose is a relatively recent addition to man's diet, man is not biochemically adapted to handling this compound well. Further, since sucrose provides calories but not other nutrients, it may lead to overeating. He also states that the correlation between sugar and myocardial infarctions is better than the correlation between fat and infarctions for individuals in a number of countries.

Epidemiological data alone are too weak to establish causation. The best one may do is to suggest that there is a correlation between two parameters. A number of studies (both human and animal) have been performed to better examine the relationship between sucrose and disease. It was found that dietary sucrose increased serum triglyceride levels substantially but had less effect on serum cholesterol. Some studies were able to show effects of dietary carbohydrate in coronary patients but not in normal volunteers. *In vitro* studies in animals have suggested that dietary carbohydrates have profound influences on lipid metabolism. Most of these effects are probably mediated through changes in the insulin/glucagon ratio. There is a substantial gap, however, between an effect on a pathway and demonstrated causation of disease.

Evaluation of the results of these studies is confounded by several factors. Usually carbohydrate in the diet was increased at the expense of fat. It then becomes impossible to differentiate effects due to higher carbohydrate levels from those due to lower fat levels. Diets comparing simple and complex carbohydrates very frequently do not have the same fiber content. Fiber content is known to change the cholesterol excretion rate from the body. Further, the time period of the study is also significant. Changing from one type of diet to another after a fast causes an exaggerated response in a number of metabolic parameters, a phenomenon known as overshooting. After a period of adaptation to a diet, there is frequently little difference in triglyceride levels, enzyme activities, and serum cholesterol values due to the type of dietary carbohydrate. The same thing is equally true for fat and cholesterol feeding studies. Thus, if studies are short term, any differences tend to be magnified; if they are long term, differences may not be apparent. Many parameters are measured in humans after a 12 hr fast; fasting itself may also tend to negate any differences normally existent in the fed state.

If one merely uses mortality rates and/or disappearance data for determining the correlation between disease states and the consumption of various dietary constituents, there are some inherent dangers in this approach as well. Mortality rates could be going down while actual disease incidence rises. Lower mortality could be the result of faster, better treatment, improved patient monitoring, etc. Disappearance data do not take into account that what is produced and purchased may not be consumed in the same form, if it is consumed at all. For example, substantial quantities of sugar might be used in the production of ethanol. Even though the sugar is still consumed, it is not consumed in the same chemical form. Consumption data for fats and oils may be even less accurate than those for carbohydrates. Much of the fat is used for frying. Although it may seem that some fast-food establishments never discard their used frying oil, in theory at least, much of the frying oil is discarded before it gets rancid. Considerable amounts of fat purchased may not actually be consumed.

With these cautions in mind, it should be noted that there is a poor correlation between sucrose consumption and heart disease deaths (Nuttall and Gannon, 1981). Further, high sucrose diets have not resulted in atherogenesis in animal studies with the exception of one rabbit study (Kritchevsky *et al.* 1968). Obesity is a strong risk factor for insulin independent (maturity onset) diabetes. To the extent that elevated sucrose consumption contributes to obesity, excess dietary sucrose may also be considered a risk factor for diabetes. There is no evidence, however, that eating sugar (in any form) causes diabetes. Once a person becomes diabetic, it is generally agreed that use of simple sugars should be considerably restricted. This precaution helps to control large swings in blood glucose levels. Consumption of complex carbohydrates need not necessarily be reduced. Indeed, consumption of complex carbohydrates actually seems to improve glucose tolerance.

Does sucrose cause obesity? It is certainly possible to induce obesity in humans and animals by providing extra calories in the form of sucrose. Anytime more calories are consumed than are used, weight gain results. Our modern way of life is largely sedentary which contributes to consumption of food in excess of need. Demonstrating that sucrose itself is an inducer of obesity is quite another matter. How might such an effect be induced? One way would be for sucrose to be a very poor inducer of the satiety response. That is, when one eats sucrose, the signal that enough has been consumed to meet energy demand might not be sent or be sent tardily. In the meantime the person continues to eat thus overconsuming calories. There is no evidence to support such a hypothesis at this time. Another possible mechanism is that sucrose (glucose + fructose) is inherently deposited as fat. Although both glucose and fructose are excellent precursors of fat, whether fat is made is more a function of the total calories and what the proportion of fat to carbohydrate is in the diet than to the type of carbohydrate. Another possibility is that sucrose consumption lowers the basal metabolic rate. The "efficiency" of the body would then be altered so that it could function on fewer calories. Therefore, continued consumption of a "normal" amount of calories would result in weight gain. Again, there is no evidence that such a mechanism exists.

B. FRUCTOSE METABOLISM

Since no sucrose enters circulation because it is broken down to glucose + fructose by sucrase in the gut, it must be assumed that any potential effects of sucrose would be mediated through either one or both monosaccharides. It is generally supposed that any potential effects of sucrose on metabolism are mediated through fructose. In a number of studies in animals, fructose was found to enhance lipogenesis to a greater degree than glucose. Activities of enzymes involved in lipogenesis rise when high sucrose or fructose diets are fed. It might reasonably be supposed that these effects are mediated through an increase in insulin levels, but fructose feeding (stomach tube) does not raise serum immunoreactive insulin levels (Cryer *et al.* 1974). If there is a distinctive effect of fructose, it is probably not exerted via insulin.

C. DENTAL CARIES

Dental caries is one disease where sucrose does indeed have an apparent causative role. Caries themselves are the result of bacterial action on a tooth. Bacteria use dietary sugars to form a mucin that adheres to the surface of a tooth and together with bacteria is called *plaque*. Then some of the dietary sugar is metabolized to acids, which together with hydrolytic bacteria destroy the tooth enamel which leads to further decay. In the absence of the offending bacteria, no cavities will result regardless of the quantity of carbohydrate in the diet. The degree to which sucrose serves as a substrate for these pathogenic bacteria (e.g., *Streptococcus mutans*) depends on the length of time the sucrose stays in proximity with the tooth. For example, taffy is far more deleterious than a less sticky food. Sucrose may not be more cariogenic than other sugars, but it is the sugar consumed in the highest amount by the general population. Therefore, it is a greater contributor to caries by virtue of its higher proportion in the diet of most people.

At this time no definitive statements can be made concerning the role of sucrose in disease with the exception of its role in caries. Sucrose is definitely a cheap source of calories and is readily shippable and storable in most locations in the world. It could be that certain subgroups in the general population are sensitive to the type and amount of dietary carbohydrate and that they develop diseases as a result of this consumption. Evidence so far suggests that this is not the case for the general population. Until such time as definitive evidence is available, advice to restrict sucrose intake would be premature and irresponsible.

D. SUMMARY

Sucrose has become widely available only in the last 200 years; before that it was available on a limited basis only to the fortunate few.

In recent years concern has been epressed that sucrose might be involved in the etiology of such diseases as dental caries, diabetes, obesity, and heart disease. To date, sucrose has been definitively shown to be causative for dental caries. To the extent that sucrose consumption contributes to overeating, it might also be said to contribute to obesity. Its role in any other syndromes has yet to be demonstrated.

REVIEW QUESTIONS

1. What is overshooting?
2. What errors are associated with using disappearance data to support correlations between certain dietary constituents and disease states?
3. Explain the role of sucrose in dental caries.

BIBLIOGRAPHY

Ahrens, R. 1974. Sucrose, hypertension and heart disease. Am. J. Clin. Nutr. *27*, 403–422.

Alling, C., Cahlin, E., and Schersten, T. 1973. Relationships between fatty acid patterns of serum, hepatic and biliary lectins in man. Biochim. Biophys. Acta *296*, 518–526.

Bibby, B. 1978. Dental caries. Caries Res. *12* Suppl. 1, 3–7.

Campbell, R., and Zinner, D. 1970. Effect of certain dietary sugars on hamster caries. J. Nutr. *100*, 14–20.

Cryer, A., Riley, S., Williams, E., and Robinson, D. 1974. Effects of fructose, sucrose, and glucose feeding on plasma insulin concentrations and on adipose tissue clearing factor lipase activity in the rat. Biochem. J. *140*, 561–563.

Geelan, M., Harris, R., Beynen, A., and McCume, S. 1980. Short-term hormonal control of hepatic lipogenesis. Diabetes *29*, 1006–1022.

Hugill, A. 1979. Sucrose—a royal carbohydrate. *In* Developments in Sweetners, Vol. 1. C. Hough, K. Parker, and A. Vlitos (Editors). Applied Science Publ., London.

Kritchevsky, D., Sallata, P., and Tepper, S. 1968. Experimental atherosclerosis in rabbits fed cholesterol-free diets. J. Atheroscler. Res. *8*, 697–703.

Nuttall, F., and Gannon, M. 1981. Sucrose and disease. Diabetes Care *4*, 305–310.

Olefsky, J., and Crapo, P. 1980. Fructose, xylitol and sorbitol. Diabetes Care *3*, 390–393.

Preuss, H., and Fournier, R. 1982. Effects of sucrose ingestion on blood pressure. Life Sci. *30*, 879–886.

Tepperman, J., and Tepperman, H. 1958. The hexose monophosphate shunt and adaptive hyperlipogenesis. Am. J. Physiol. *193*, 55–64.

Yudkin, J. 1963. Nutrition and palatability with special reference to obesity, myocardial infarction and other diseases of civilization. The Lancet *1*, June 22, 1335–1338.

Part V

Industrial Uses of Carbohydrates

17

Sweeteners

Most of the world's population values sweet taste. Many people say a meal is not complete until they have had a taste of something sweet. Our social functions often revolve around the serving of an assortment of sweet foods: pies, cakes, cookies, and candy. Even terms of affection and endearment reflect our sweet tooth: "honey," "sweetheart," and "sugar."

Although sweeteners are readily available today such has not always been the case. Until the nineteenth century, only the very wealthy could afford to indulge a craving for sweets. The rest of the population had to make do with the use of fruit and occasionally honey. The early history of sweeteners has been reviewed by Hugill (1979). Use of sweeteners is not a modern concept because early cave drawings indicate a man robbing a bees' nest. Beekeeping was known to the ancient Egyptians. Use of sugar cane for sucrose, however, was probably a later development. The very early history of sugar cane is uncertain but its earliest cultivation may have started in Oceania. Most of the earliest references to it in Western literature discuss its use in Persia and India. Sugar did not reach England until the 1300s, but is was very rare and exorbitantly expensive. The price did not really decline much until the iniquitous slave trade provided a source of inexpensive labor to produce sugar in the colonies. The 1800s brought the development of a commercially feasible sugar beet technology and prices declined still further.

There can be too much of a good thing. For much of his history man has engaged in ways to acquire sweeteners. Now that they are readily available and cheap, he is again not satisfied. He must have something that tastes sweet without adding calories. In the past several decades considerable attention has been given to the production of "nonnutritive" sweeteners. To be useful these compounds must be at least as sweet as sucrose with properties that do not alter the texture or appearance of food. If they are not compatible with the normal physical properties of foods, then they must be many times sweeter than sucrose so that their addition will be in very small amounts. Nonnutritive sweeteners must, of course, be safe to use and economical to produce.

A. Nutritive Sweeteners

By definition the nutritive sweeteners are those compounds that taste sweet and contain calories. They include table sugar (sucrose), glucose (dextrose), fructose, galactose, lactose, maltose, xylitol, and sorbitol. They may also be mixtures of carbohydrates such as are found in corn syrup, honey, maple syrup, or molasses.

Sucrose may be refined from sugar cane or sugar beets. Another development which contributed substantially to the availability of sweeteners was the production of syrup from starch. Early syrup was produced from partial acid hydrolysis of corn or potato starch and was composed of a mixture of glucose, maltose, and other saccharides. Sucrose production (cane and beet) in the 1970s was about 80×10^6 tons/year whereas D-glucose and syrup production was 10×10^6 tons/year. Since less than 10% of the U.S. corn crop is used for syrup production, this ensures a stable, low-cost supply of raw material. Even in years when the corn production is down substantially, there is an adequate supply for corn syrup production.

Cane sugar production relies on the successful growing of the reedy perennial cane plant. It grows well only in a 25° latitude range on either side of the equator where the climate is warm but with distinct wet and dry seasons. Such restrictive conditions limit to a large extent where cane can be readily grown. Sugar cane is host for a number of fungal and parasitic pests and deteriorates rapidly after cutting due to bacterial spoilage. In modern cane sugar mills the cut cane is chopped, the juice is extracted with hot water, and then treated with lime to precipitate contaminants and vacuum dried to get the sucrose crystals. The mother syrup is again subjected to crystalization leaving a final syrup called black-strap molasses, which has a number of important commercial uses including production of alcoholic beverages and cattle feed.

Production of beet sugar has some advantage in that sugar beets grow nicely in temperate climates. Since the beet is an annual it offers the further advantage of being rotatable with other crops to prevent soil depletion. After being mechanically harvested, sugar beets are cut into thin slices and the juice is extracted with hot water. The rest of the refining process is very similar to that used for cane sugar although different impurities are found in the raw sugar from the two sources. Following refining, however, the final products are virtually indistinguishable.

The technology of corn syrup production has been outlined in an excellent review by MacAllister (1979). The most common corn syrup in this country is 42 D.E. (dextrose equivalent) (100 parts of syrup is equal in reducing power to 42 parts of D-glucose). This syrup is made by acid hydrolysis of corn starch. Although the theoretical yield is 111 D.E., rarely are syrups above 55 D.E. manufactured because undesirable flavors are produced that are difficult to remove economically. To be called a syrup, a product must have dextrose equivalent of at least 20.

The steps of corn syrup processing are outlined in Fig. 17.1. First the corn is wet-milled to separate the kernel into its constituent parts. This process yields starch at very high purity (99%). A slurry of the starch is then pumped to a converter where it is boiled with hydrochloric acid under pressure until a 42 D.E. syrup is attained (6 min at 45 psi). The contents of the converter are ejected and neutralized with sodium carbonate. Protein material flocculates and is filtered out at this point and fatty contaminantes are readily skimmed off. Both can be used in animal feeds. The neutralized extract is then concentrated by evaporation and treated with activated carbon to remove contaminants. The final step is further evaporation to yield a product with 82% solids. The steps are outlined in Fig. 17.1.

Crystalline glucose (dextrose) can also be made from starch. Originally glucose was prepared from 90 D.E. syrups obtained by acid hydrolysis of starch using a high proportion of nucleating glucose seed crystals and agitation of the liquor. Now, however, the starting material is obtained by enzymatic rather than acid hydrolysis of starch.

Use of enzymes lessens processing costs because they work at neutral pH's and atmospheric pressure eliminating the need for expensive high pressure, noncorrosive processing systems. Enzymatic treatment also results in fewer undesirable reaction products. One of the most used enzymes is bacterial α-*amylase,* an endoamylase that cleaves starch at interior parts of the chain. β-*amylase* can also be used. This is an examylase and works from the nonreducing end of the starch chain. β-Amylase, however, converts starch only to maltose unless there are α(1,6) branch points where its action is blocked. *Glucoamylase* also attacks starch from the nonreducing end releasing D-glucose. It also can cleave α(1→6) bonds but at a much slower rate than α(1→4) bonds. To effectively cleave these α(1→6) bonds *pullinase* can be used. *Iso-*

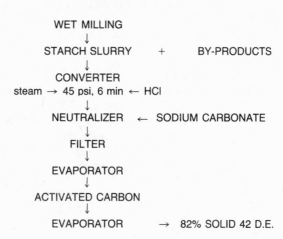

WET MILLING
↓
STARCH SLURRY   +   BY-PRODUCTS
↓
CONVERTER
steam → 45 psi, 6 min ← HCl
↓
NEUTRALIZER   ← SODIUM CARBONATE
↓
FILTER
↓
EVAPORATOR
↓

FIG. 17.1. Block diagram   ACTIVATED CARBON
of the production of 42 D.E.   ↓
corn syrup.   EVAPORATOR   →   82% SOLID 42 D.E.

amylse is also active against (1→6) bonds but its specificity is for units of at least three glucosyl residues attached via an α(1→6) link to the rest of the chain.

Enzyme reactors made by immobilizing enzymes of the appropriate type on some solid support may be used for starch hydrolysis. The substrate is passed through the column reactors to achieve the desired reactions. This method has the advantage of eliminating the need to remove the enzymes from the final product by some denaturing technique. This saves a processing step and in effect makes the enzymes reusable.

Glucose can be converted to other sugars as well. One of the chief conversions is glucose to fructose, a process that is predominately enzymatic although conversions can also be achieved chemically. Bacterial isomerases (which have a metal ion requirement) are used. This technology is employed in the production of high fructose corn syrups. These syrups are useful because under some conditions they are sweeter; therefore, less is needed. Since fructose does not readily crystallize out, such syrups can be concentrated to a greater extent than glucose syrups. Thus volumes and shipping costs are reduced. Crystalline fructose may be made from fructose syrups with judicious selection of processing parameters. The conventional commercial procedure is to crystallize the fructose from a water/alcohol mixture.

Fructose technology is advancing rapidly because of the increasing emphasis on the use of fructose as an alternative to sucrose. There is still debate concerning the general use of fructose. Although fructose was at one time touted as a sweetener suitable for diabetics, there has been a reexamination of this premise. Some studies have implicated fructose in hypertriglyceridemia but these effects may be transient.

Fructose has the advantage over some sweeteners in that it leaves no bitter aftertaste and is suitable for boiling, baking, canning, and freezing. It has a good shelf life in baked products. In the cold, at acid pH's fructose is sweeter than sucrose so less can be used. It is also sweeter than sorbitol and about as sweet as xylitol. Sugar sweetness has been ranked by Moskowitz (1971,1974) in the following order fructose > xylitol > sucrose > glucose > mannitol > lactose > maltose = sorbitol.

Sorbitol, another commonly used nutritive sweetener, is found in plants and is relatively economical to produce commercially. The drawback to sorbitol is that it is only about one-fourth as sweet as fructose. Further, since it enters the body from the gut by passive diffusion, it can cause osmotic diarrhea when consumed in amounts over 30 g/day. Ingestion apparently does not lead to intracellular sorbitol accumulation. Although sorbitol certainly can be transformed into glucose in normal metabolic pathways, its entry into the body is slow enough so that it does not lead to a rise in blood glucose.

When introduced commercially, xylitol was expected to be a huge success in the nutritive sweetener market. Xylitol is noncariogenic and therefore a boon to those wishing to save their teeth. It can cause osmotic diarrhea, but there is little problem in this regard if quantities are restricted. It was found, however, that xylitol could cause bladder tumors in mice when ingested at high levels. Rather than to embark on expensive and possibly inconclusive studies to prove its safety, food manufacturers have ceased using xylitol as a nutritive sweetener.

B. NONNUTRITIVE SWEETENERS

Nonnutritive sweeteners are those compounds that provide a high degree of sweetness but have little or no caloric value. Saccharin, cyclamate, aspartame, the dihydrochalcones, and glycyrrhizin are in this category (Fig. 17.2). Monellin, a 10,000 MW protein, might also be considered to belong to this group because although proteins are caloric, monellin is about 2000 times sweeter than sucrose so only very small amounts would be needed. Consequently, it would provide almost no calories.

Saccharin is the oldest of the nonnutritive sweeteners having been synthesized in 1879 by Remsen and Fahlberg (Kalkhoff and Levin 1978). Depending on the standard against which it is measured, sac-

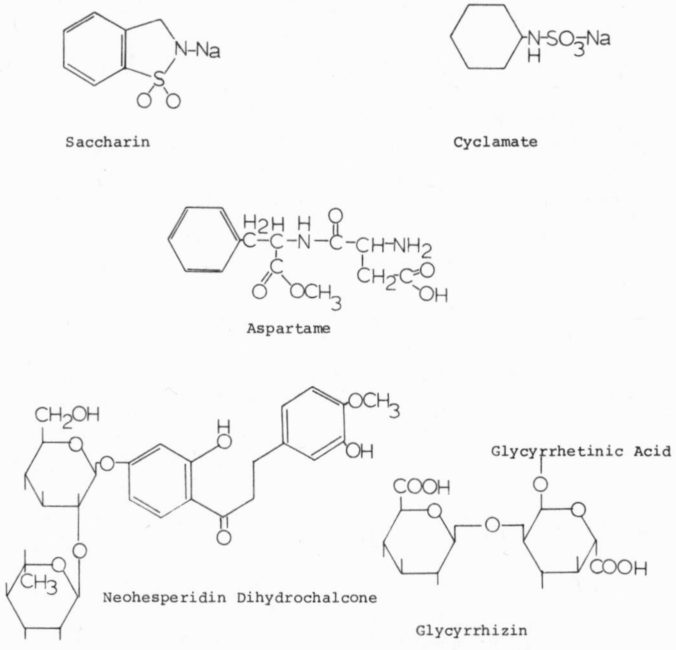

FIG. 17.2.   Structures of the nonnutritive sweeteners.

charin is from 200 to 700 times sweeter than sucrose. It is frequently used as a diet aid, and as an additive to cosmetics, prescription, and over-the-counter drugs. A large part of saccharin consumption is in the form of low calorie soft drinks. Saccharin was popular during World War II when sugar was scarce. The popularity of saccharin decreased when cyclamates were introduced, but when cyclamates were banned, saccharin enjoyed a resurgence of popularity.

Saccharin is not metabolized or stored in the human. Studies have shown that 90% of a labeled dose is recovered within 48 hr in the urine. A small amount is excreted in the feces and trace amounts can be recovered in the bile. Studies with pregnant monkeys suggest that saccharin is transferrable across the placenta and that fetal clearance is considerably slower than maternal clearance.

Commercial saccharin may contain impurities ranging from 40 to 7000 ppm. Care is necessary in interpreting studies on effects of saccharin because some studies have been performed with grossly impure preparations. Kalkhoff and Levin (1971) have reviewed the studies concerning the carcinogenicity and mutagenicity of saccharin. They noted that a variety of exerimental methods have shown the compound to be carcinogenic but that many other investigators using the same techniques have been unable to reproduce the effects. Similarly, mutagenicity studies have failed to yield clear, reproducible results. Based on modified Ames testing and saccharin preparations of varying purity, it has been found that only pure preparations were nonmutagenic. In human epidemiological studies, only one out of many studies (several of which screened 20,000 patients) found any link between bladder cancer and saccharin use. Further, although saccharin use was higher among diabetic patients than in nondiabetics, this subpopulation had no greater incidence of bladder cancer than the controls. Neither animal nor human studies to date have provided unequivocal evidence about the risks involved in saccharin use. Many studies in animals have used amounts of this sweetener which are far in excess of usual consumption. This also needs to be taken into account in evaluating potential risk of saccharin use.

On the plus side are the advantages to diabetics and obese persons of having a palatable nonnutritive sweetener to replace sugar. The risks of being obese or diabetic are more well defined and the consequences of sucrose use in these individuals are better understood than the risk of developing cancer from nonnutritive sweeteners. One must balance, therefore, the risk entailed with potential benefits. The Food and Drug Administration planned to ban saccharin use. Since cyclamate had been banned earlier and no other nonnutritive sweetener was available, public outcry succeeded in delaying the ban. Products containing saccharin, however, must carry a warning on the label about a potential health hazard.

Cyclamate was discovered to be sweet by Sveda at the University of Illinois in 1937. Use of cyclamate as a sweetener was approved by the

Food and Drug Administration in 1950. Cyclamate is only 30 times sweeter than sucrose. Saccharin is far sweeter but leaves an unpleasant aftertaste. For this reason, after 1953 cyclamate and saccharin were mixed in a 10 to 1 ratio to optimize taste and sweetness of food and drinks.

Like saccharin, cyclamate enters and leaves the body essentially unchanged. Less than 1% of the dose is metabolized to cyclohexylamine. In 1969, results of a 2 year animal study led to the ban of cyclamate by the FDA. Although the study was not designed as a carcinogenicity experiment, a higher incidence of bladder tumors were found in cyclamate fed animals. Subsequent studies have been unable to confirm the early results, but the ban has never been lifted.

A newer possibility for a nonnutritive sweetener is the dipeptide *aspartame,* composed of aspartate and phenylalanine methyl ester which is about 200 times sweeter than sucrose. Although aspartame is caloric, so little is required for use that essentially no calories are added. The compound is unstable in aqueous solution, so its use will likely be restricted to dehydrated foods. Aspartame was approved for use in 1974 but never marketed. In 1980, approval was withdrawn based on three studies suggesting that aspartame was carcinogenic. Since aspartame fed at high doses would presumably contribute to an amino acid imbalance, the results from the usual methods of tumor testing using high doses may not be valid. In 1981, the FDA again approved aspartame for use in spite of continued concern about its safety (Smith 1981).

Sweeteners produced from *naringen* (found in citrus fruit peels) hold some promise for the future. Neohesperidin dihydrocalcone is most likely to be the agent of choice. Although it is 300 times sweeter than sucrose, the onset of sweet taste is slower but lingers longer than that of sucrose. Where other flavors are present in a food that needs to be balanced by simultaneous sweetening, there is a strong disadvantage to use of this sweetener because bitter and sour tastes would be perceived first. In some products, such as chewing gum, however, slow onset of sweet taste would be an advantage.

Glycyrrihizin is 50 times sweeter than sucrose. This compound comes from the same shrub as licorice flavoring. It is found primarily in the roots of the plant which grows in the Orient, Russia, and southern Europe. Glycyrrhizin is produced by crystallization from extracts of the roots. It is on the GRAS (generally recognized as safe) list of the FDA.

Monellin is far sweeter than any of the other currently known nonnutritive sugar substitutes. Since it is a 10,000 MW peptide it really does have calories. At that sweetening power, however, so little would be used that negligible calories would be added to a food. Such low levels of use might also limit toxicologic problems. Monellin is isolated from the berries of the West African plant, *Dioscoreophyllum cumminisii.* Originally, it was erroneously characterized as a carbohydrate owing probably to the difficulty of separating the peptide from the berry mucilage. Commercial development of this compound has been of limited interest because it is unstable to heat and low pH. Monellin, however, has been a useful tool in the investigation of the perception of sweet taste. It is interesting to note that monellin only tastes sweet to man and Old World monkeys; other animals that ordinarily perceive other sweet tastes do not respond to monellin. Insufficient data exist for this sweetener to be deemed safe by the FDA.

A number of health impairing conditions such as obesity and diabetes demand that alternatives to sucrose be found. The alternatives must be safe and have an acceptable sweetness without an objectionable aftertaste. Their properties should not interfere with the physical properties of the food to which they are added.

C. SUMMARY

Wide availability of sugar is a development of the last two centuries. Before that, sweeteners were available only to the very wealthy or to those lucky enough to have access to a beehive. Modern technology has made available sugars and syrups from cane and sugar beets and from corn starch. Sweeteners can be divided into two groups: nutritive and nonnutritive. The nutritive ones, such as sucrose, glucose, fructose, and the polyols, provide calories whereas the nonnutritive ones, such as saccharin, cyclamate, dihydrochalcone, aspartame, or monellin, are calorie free either by virtue of their nonmetabolizability or the very small amounts in which they are used. The nonnutritive sweetener represent a number of chemical categories including glycosides, dipeptides, and proteins. Not all of these have properties that are desirable for every application.

REVIEW QUESTIONS

1. What are nonnutritive sweeteners?
2. What two different processes can be used to produce corn syrups from cornstarch?
3. Why is high fructose corn syrup desirable?

BIBLIOGRAPHY

Crosby, G., and Wingard, R.   1979.   A survey of less common sweeteners. *In* Developments in Sweeteners, Vol. 1. C. Hough, K. Parker, and A. Vlitos (Editors). Applied Science Publ., London.
Daniels, R.   1973.   Sugar Substitutes and Enhancers. Noyes Data Corp., Park Ridge, New Jersey.
Higginbotham, J.   1979.   Protein sweeteners. *In* Development in Sweeteners, Vol. 1. C. Hough, K. Parker, and A. Vlitos (Editors). Applied Sci. Publ., London.

Hugill, A. 1979. Sucrose—a royal carbohydrate. *In* Developments in Sweeteners, Vol. 1. C. Hough, K. Parker, and A. Vlitos (Editors). Applied Sci. Publ., London.

Kalkhoff, R., and Levin, M. 1978. The saccharin controversy. Diabetes Care *1*, 211–222.

MacAllister, R. 1979. Nutritive sweeteners made from starch. Adv. Carbohydr. Chem. Biochem. *36*, 15–56.

Mazur, R., and Ripper, A. 1979. Peptide-based sweeteners. *In* Developments in Sweeteners, Vol. 1. C. Hough, K. Parker, and A. Vlitos (Editors). Applied Science Publ., London

Moskowitz, O. 1971. The sweetness and pleasantness of sugars. Am. J. Psychol. *84*, 387–405.

Moskowitz, O. 1974. The psychology of sugars. *In* Sugars in Nutrition. H. Sipple and K. McNutt (Editors). Academic Press, New York.

Smith, R. 1981. Aspartame approved despite risks. Science *213*, 986–987.

18

Alcohol

Alcoholic fermentation has been carried on purposefully or accidently for many centuries. It was not until the eighteenth century, however, that Spallanzani suggested that fermentation was casually related to microbial growth. In 1837, Cagniard-Latour, Schwann, and Kutzing independently proposed that yeast was responsible for alcohol production. This theory was severely attacked by a number of reputable chemists of the time, including Liebig and Wohler, who believed that fermentation was a purely chemical process. The biggest advances in the understanding of fermentation came from Pasteur in the mid-1800s. Pasteur also showed that the end products of fermentation are dependent on the specific microorganism.

Production of ethyl alcohol is an important industrial process. In excess of 500 million gallons of industrial alcohol are produced per year in the United States, and much of this is obtained by fermentation processes. Production of alcoholic beverages entails quite different concerns than production for industrial use. For beverages, taste, color, and odor of the end products are more important than cost of starting materials. Raw materials cost is, however, a primary concern in production of industrial alcohol. Molasses, barley, potatoes, and corn have all been extensively used as the carbohydrate source for the making of alcohol. In light of the energy crisis there has been increasing interest in the production of ethanol from biomass to use as a fuel source to spare fossil reserves of oil and gas.

In order to be useful, ethanol production from the biomass must be energy efficient; the ethanol must replace more fuel than its production uses. Its production also should not use up the supplies of premium oil-based fuels.

A. NATURAL FERMENTATIONS (BEVERAGES)

Regardless of the type of alcoholic beverage, production relies on a source of fermentable carbohydrate. This may be a simple carbohydrate as in the case of wine making or a complex carbohydrate such as barley starches in beer manufacture. The taste of the final product may also depend in part on the addition of other agents such as hops for

TABLE 18.1. Use of Grains for Beverage
Alcohol Use[a]

Grain	Millions of bushels	
	1975	1980
Corn	71.1	73
Barley	124.8	160 (estimate)
Sorghum	2.8	4.0

[a] Data obtained from USDA publication "Feed-Out-look and Situation" Feb. 1981.

beer or the use of charred oak barrels for various whiskeys. Corn, barley, and sorghum are used in considerable quantities for beverage alcohol production in the United States. Consumption data are shown in Table 18.1. The use of 73 million bushels of corn for alcohol production should be compared to a total annual corn harvest of approximately 8 billion bushels. The percentage of the barley crop which goes into alcoholic beverages is higher than that for corn. Barley has little gluten content making it unsuitable for baking. Thus there is not a strong competition for this grain by another industry. Barley germinates readily and has a protected sprout. This grain has a strong outer husk and is relatively resistant to molds which is an advantage over huskless grains such as wheat. The husks also aid in the filtration steps of the brewing process.

The United States is the world's leading producer of beer (Jackson 1977) (about 180 hectoliters/year in 1977) followed by West Germany, which produces less than half of the U.S. amount. West Germany, however, consumes nearly twice as much beer per capita as the United States. Most countries produce some form of beer even though they may not have a flourishing brewing industry.

There are three general categories of beer: top-fermented, top-fermented containing wheat, and bottom-fermented. These classifications are not very specific, and there is not general agreement throughout the world that such terminology should be used. The method of fermenting grain in the brewing of beer is much like the fermentation process for producing industrial alcohol. The difference is that great care is taken at each step to regulate color, odor, and taste since the ethanol will not be distilled away from by-products of the fermentation reactions.

The general process consists of turning the grain into a malt, adding the hops for flavor and preservation, and adding yeast to cause fermentation. The first process in beer making when barley is used is the malting of the grain. To allow solubilization of the starches in barley, which has a very hard covering, the grain is germinated in a controlled fashion; the process is terminated by drying. At this point the grain may be roasted to impart special flavors and colors to the beer. The barley is then finely ground and other grains may be added. These others grains must be precooked to solubilize the starch.

The next step is to produce mash by adding hot water to the ground grain to convert starches into fermentable sugars. The mash is filtered and the spent grains may be further processed for animal feeds. The clarified mash, called *wort*, is then heated to boiling to sterilize it. This step may be accomplished by pressurized steam or by direct fire on the kettles (fire-brewed beer). Next carrageenan from red algae may be added to clarify the wort. Hops are also added at this point.

A number of plants have been used to impart taste, clarity, crispness, and preservative qualities to beer. Among these are hops, junipers, bay, and coriander. Hops are most commonly used today. They may be added as the natural flower or as a pelleted form or as an extract (less popular). The flower is found only on female plants, and it is preferable that the flower not be fertilized because hop seeds are a nuisance in the brewing process. The hop flower contains yellow glands, which yield tannins, resins, essential oils, and α acids (humulones) crucial to the beermaking. The humulones have a secondary function as a preservative and antiseptic.

Fermentation is the next step. For bottom-fermented beer, fermentation is accomplished at cool temperatues. There is a primary stage, lasting a week, and a secondary stage called variously aging, conditioning, ripening, or lagering. The second stage occurs at very cool temperatures and may last several months. During this time there is some secondary fermentation of the more inaccessible sugars. After this stage the beer is filtered.

For top-fermented beer, the fermentation process is considerably shorter. The primary fermentation is accomplished at higher temperatures. The secondary phase requires only a few days. During this phase sugar is added to stimulate secondary fermentation, and the beer is placed into casks which are sealed to allow CO_2 to build up providing carbonation.

Beer that is going to be stored for some time following fermentation is pasteurized. Although pasteurization improves shelf life, it does lead to some loss of taste and carbonation. Preservatives are added to some beers to extend their life. Beers that are not pasteurized must be consumed within a short time after manufacture.

Wine making is essentially similar to the process for making beer. Instead of starting with complex carbohydrates that one finds in grains, however, the carbohydrates that serve as substrates for fermentation are mostly glucose and fructose found in grape juice. The juices are sterilized, inoculated with a desirable strain of yeast, and aerated to promote active yeast growth. Next the conditions are made anaerobic so that alcohol rather than CO_2 and water is produced. The strains of yeast used in wine making will produce 7–15% alcohol. The degree of sweetness or dryness of the wine is determined by the extent to which the fermentation is allowed to proceed. Bottling before fermentation is complete allows carbonation from CO_2 production to produce a sparkling wine. If the fermentation is completed before bottling then the product is a still wine. Addition of extra alcohol leads to fortified wines such as sherry and port (16–35% alcohol).

Brandy is essentially distilled wine, a process that greatly increases the alcohol content. Bourbon is distilled from a fermented mash that contained at least 51% corn. Like beer, scotch whiskey comes from a fermented barley malt. Whiskey is the generic term for a beverage containing 43–50% alcohol distilled from a mixture of malts of corn, barley, and rye.

B. ALCOHOL FOR INDUSTRIAL/COMMERCIAL USE

The increasing interest in alcohol as a fuel (gasohol) has lent impetus to the development of a number of small and large scale plants for alcohol production from biomass. Regardless of the system there are three basic steps involved: (1) formation of a fermentable sugar (saccharification), (2) fermentation of the sugar to alcohol, and (3) distillation of the alcohol to purify it from other components of the system. The overall process using corn as a starting material is outlined in Fig. 18.1. The initial steps may vary depending on the starting material. If the material is starch from grain, the starch must first be exposed by finely grinding the grain and then hydrated to render it susceptible to attack by amylases to form glucose. During this portion of the processing a sufficiently high temperature is attained to "sterilize" the mash thus contaminating microorganisms are destroyed and unwanted side reactions are prevented. Once the simple sugars are produced, then the next phase can begin. If the starting material contains sugars instead of starch, then only a sugar extraction process is needed before fermentation can begin.

Fermentation is accomplished by inoculating the mash with brewers' yeast (*Saccharomyces cerevisiae*), which produces ethanol anaerobically from glucose (or fructose). Ethanol will not reach a concentration

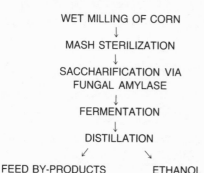

FIG. 18-1. Process for producing ethanol from corn.

much above 9% at this stage because the microorganisms are killed by the ethanol. Theoretically, for each 100 lb of sugar fermented, 7.7 gallons of ethanol (51 lb) and 49 lb of carbon dioxide are produced. In addition, there are also small amounts of contaminants produced such as fusel oil, succinate, and glycerol. The time required for maximum fermentation to occur is dependent on the strain of yeast. Some yeasts are far more efficient than others. Care must be taken during fermentation to exclude oxygen and vent the carbon dioxide since fermentation is an anaerobic process. The final step is the distillation process where the ethanol is removed from the mash and concentrated. The residue, consisting of residual grain and spent yeast, can be used for animal feeds.

This process can be extended to using cellulose as a starting material. Wood chips, plant wastes, or municipal paper wastes might serve as the starting material. A different depolymerization method is required in order to break cellulose down to carbohydrate monomers. A high degree of lignification may hamper this breakdown process. One process presently in use, according to a TRW report (1980) employs enzymes from a mutant strain of *Trichoderma reesei*. In this scheme saccharification and fermentation occur in the same step. The TRW report states that municipal solid waste would be an acceptable source of cellulose for this process.

Several other systems utilizing cellulose have been described but are not yet scaled up to production levels. One is being developed at the University of Pennsylvania in conjunction with General Electric (Paul 1980). The starting material undergoes dilute acid hydrolysis with sulfur dioxide before enzyme treatment. Most of the SO_2 can be recovered, minimizing waste disposal difficulties, but the process is very corrosive. An alternative technology, also being developed at the University of Pennsylvania, delignifies the cellulose with aqueous butanol. Separation of the solubilized lignin from the sugars represents a formidable task.

After the ethanol is obtained, special precautions must be taken. Ethanol is very volatile and has a low flash point (55°C). Proper storage must include fire safety measures. Ethanol is also very hydroscopic. Absorption of water from the air lowers the proof of the alcohol and makes it less useful as a fuel (less than 192 proof will not work for use in gasohol).

To avoid the possibility of using industrial alcohol for beverage purposes, denaturants are added. There are several formulas but one (CDA 19) is constituted as follows: 100 gallons ethanol + 4 gallons methylisobutyl ketone + 1 gallon kerosene. Denatured alcohol is unfit for human consumption and unrecoverable as a beverage.

The impact of major use of ethanol produced from corn on U.S. agriculture has been calculated. If ethanol were used for gasohol in a 1 to 10 ratio with gasoline, then 10^9 gallons/year of ethanol would be required by 1990. Such an amount would necessitate the additional production of 4×10^9 bushels of corn per year, a nearly 50% increase in the present corn harvest.

C. SUMMARY

Alcoholic fermentation of carbohydrate is an important process for the manufacture of alcoholic beverages and industrial alcohols. The processes involved are essentially alike except that by-products are of greater concern in beverage alcohol making whereas raw material costs are most important for industrial alcohol. The first step in the process is to obtain fermentable sugars. Wine making starts with sugars in the form of grape juice. When grains are used (as in beer and whiskey making), it is necessary to break down the starch, usually in an enzymatic process. Next fermentation occurs, then some form of aging process for beer and wine followed by bottling. Industrial alcohol or distilled spirits manufacture requires a distillation step after fermentation. Depending on the type of beverage, further aging may also be needed after distillation. Increasing efforts are being made to find economical ways to make industrial alcohol because of its potential for use as an alternate energy source. Although presently only in the pilot plant stage, processes to convert municipal cellulosic wastes promise considerable potential for industrial alcohol production.

REVIEW QUESTIONS

1. What advantage does barley offer as a starting material for the beer production?
2. What is the difference in still and sparkling wine and how is it brought about?
3. What is the theoretical yield of ehtanol from 100 lbs of sugar?
4. Define saccharification.

BIBLIOGRAPHY

Anon. 1980. Energy balances in the production and end-use of alcohols derived from biomass. TRW Energy Systems Planning Division for U.S. Dept. of Energy.
Jackson, M. (Editor). 1977. The World Guide to Beer. Ballentine Books, New York.
Paul, J. (Editor). 1980. Large and Small Scale Ethyl Alcohol Manufacturing Processes from Agricultural Raw Materials. Noyes Data Corp., Park Ridge, New Jersey.

19

Specialized Uses of Carbohydrates

Certain types of polysaccharides by virtue of their physical properties find enormous application as gums and mucilages. These compounds are high molecular weight polymers of monosaccharides hooked together in glycosidic linkages. When suspended in water the polymers hydrate to form very viscous gels or mucilages. The biggest use of gums is as stabilizers (25%) and thickeners (23%) but gums are also used as film formers, agents of water retention, coagulants, colloids, and lubricants. The use of gums has increased steadily in recent years, particularly the use of gums of microbial origin. One of the biggest nonfood uses for gums is in the oil drilling and recovery industry: in 1980 an estimated 3000 tons of xanthan gum was used for this purpose. In his excellent review on microbial polysaccharides, Sandford (1979) lists the various types of common gums and their distribution of use between food and industrial use. A portion of that information is shown in Table 19.1. The applications for gums appear unlimited if gums can be found that are readily available and have appropriate properties.

The natural gums may be of plant or microbial origin. Plant gums

TABLE 19.1.   Food and Industrial Use of Natural Gums[a]

Gum	Source	Millions of pounds		
		Food	Industrial	Total
Corn starch	Seeds	600	2500	3100
Carboxymethyl cellulose	Wood pulp	16	100	116
Guar	Seeds	20	45	65
Methyl cellulose	Wood pulp	2	53	55
Arabic	Bark exudate	24	7	31
Alginate	Algae	10	2	12
Locust bean	Seeds	9	3	12
Pectin	Fruit peels	12	0	12
Xanthan	Microorganisms	3	9	12

[a] Adapted from Sanford (1979).

may be derived either from intracellular locations such as in seed coats (locust bean gum) or from extracellular exudates resulting from injury to the organism (gum arabic). Like gums from plants, microbial polysaccharides may also be of intra- or extracellular origin. Those of extracellular origin have been most used because they are easier to purify. Some care has to be exercised, however, concerning the selection of the microorganisms because many microbial exopolysaccharides are toxic to humans.

A. Galactomannans, Glucomannans, and Mannans

The galactomannans, especially, have been consumed as food since very early times. They have also become important in a number of industrial processes, and for medicinal uses. Galactomannans are linear β-mannans with single branches of α-galactose. The ratio of mannose to galactose is dependent on the source. For example, guar has a ratio of mannose to galactose of 2:1 whereas the ratio in locust bean gum from carob is from 3:1 to 6:1.

$$\alpha\text{-}D\text{-Gal}\qquad\qquad\qquad \alpha\text{-}D\text{-Gal}$$
$$\downarrow (1\rightarrow6)\qquad\qquad\qquad \downarrow (1\rightarrow6)$$
$$\beta\text{-}D\text{-Man}(1\rightarrow4)\ \beta\text{-}D\text{-Man}(1\rightarrow4)\ \beta\text{-}D\text{-Man}(1\rightarrow4)\ \beta\text{-}D\text{-Man}(1\rightarrow4)$$

Guar gum

$$\alpha\text{-}D\text{-Gal}\qquad\qquad\qquad\qquad\qquad \alpha\text{-}D\text{-Gal}$$
$$\downarrow (1\rightarrow6)\qquad\qquad\qquad\qquad\qquad \downarrow (1\rightarrow6)$$
$$\beta\text{-}D\text{-Man}(1\rightarrow4)\ \beta\text{-}D\text{-Man}(1\rightarrow4)\ \beta\text{-}D\text{-Man}(1\rightarrow4)\ \beta\text{-}D\text{-Man}(1\rightarrow4)\ \beta\text{-}D\text{-Man}(1\rightarrow4)$$

Locust bean gum

The degree of branching alters the physical properties: guar easily hydrates in cold water whereas locust bean gum must be heated in water to hydrate. Grinding of gums hastens swelling time and hydration. However, the rate may become so rapid that lumps may form which consist of fully hydrated gel on the outside with dried gel on the inside. These lumps remain stable and constitute a processing problem. This problem can be overcome to some extent by hydrating the gum in aqueous solutions of water and organic solvents such as ethyl alcohol or glycerol. Hydration is more uniformly accomplished when the aqueous solvent is sprayed into an air suspension of the finely divided gum particles.

Milling of gums also produces another undesirable characteristic, a beany odor. This is definitely objectionable when the gums are to be added to foods or cosmetics. The odor can be removed if the seeds are treated with steam before grinding. The time required for treatment is proportional to the intensity of the odor.

Guar and locust bean gums are particularly useful as food additives because they produce smooth texture and have good heat stability. Products containing guar or locust bean gums are not stringy or gelatinous and do not have a tendency to weep. The usual concentration to these gums in a product is from 3 to 8%.

Glucomannans are found in association with cellulose in woody plants. The most prevalent food source is konnyaku powder prepared from the tubers of the plant *Amorphophalis konyac*. This in turn is processed to yield konjac mannan which is a $\beta(1\rightarrow4)$ glucomannan with β-D-glucose interspersed with sequences of three mannoses.

$$\beta\text{-D-Man}(1\rightarrow4)\beta\text{-D-Man}(1\rightarrow4)\beta\text{-D-Man}(1\rightarrow4)\beta\text{-D-Glu}(1\rightarrow4)\beta\text{-D-Man}$$

In nature, pure mannans are very rare. The most frequent source is from the yeast *Saccharomyces cerevisiae* which produces an $\alpha(1\rightarrow3)$ $\alpha(1\rightarrow6)$ branched chain mannan. Short polymers of mannans are, of course, quite common on glycoproteins. There are also a number of mannose containing heteropolymers where N-acetylglucosamine is frequently the other monosaccharide in the polymer.

Since various gums are often used in foods, it is necessary to know to what extent they are digestible and how the body metabolizes any products that might be formed. Usually it is assumed that no significant digestion of mannans occurs. This may not necessarily be the case. α-Mannosidase has been detected in the GI tracts of the sheep, ox, pig, rabbit, rat, and monkey. The enzyme may be Zn^{2+} dependent and seems to have an acid pH optimum. Although mannans are not readily attacked by α-mannosidase, they are by other exo- and endomannanases.

If mannans are digested to some extent, the mannose would be passively absorbed by the gut. Once in circulation, mannose is metabolized nearly as readily as glucose and is phosphorylated to mannose 6-phosphate by hexokinase. It is next converted to fructose 6-phosphate by a Zn^{2+} containing isomerase that is distinct from glucose phosphate isomerase. Mannose 6-phosphate can also be converted to mannose 1-phosphate. This is a very important reaction because the product reacts with GTP to form GDPmannose which is the substrate for transferases which form mannose containing glycoproteins and glycolipids. GDP mannose can also be converted to GDP fucose, another important biological carbohydrate. Mannose can be converted to liver glycogen although not as efficiently as glucose. Orally administered mannose does not result in a rise in blood glucose levels because it is so slowly absorbed, and it is not found in the general circulation because it is very efficiently scavenged out of the portal circulation by the liver. Mannose stimulates insulin secretion, and insulin secretion in turn stimulates liver mannose metabolism.

The body apparently catabolizes the mannans existing on its own glycoproteins by α- and β-mannosidases from the lysosomes. Whether dietary mannans serve as a nutrient sources is still an open question.

The galactomannans and glucomannans do have hypocholes-
terolemic properties. In animal studies, these products have been
shown to interfere with reabsorption of bile. Since bile excretion is the
major route of cholesterol elimination from the body, the hypocholes-
terolemic properties of the mannans are not surprising. Two properties
are necessary for this effect: water solubility and high viscosity. When
either of these properties is altered, the gum no longer acts as a hypoc-
holesterolemic agent.

Some studies have reported that these gums reduce growth in young
animals, but these results have not been uniformly reproducible. However, an increased weight of the cecum is usually observed with diets
containing relatively high levels (5%) of guar or locust bean gums.

The mannans, when introduced *into* the body, are stimulators of
interferon production and inhibitors of tumor growth. Since polysaccharides are highly antigenic, it is possible that these two phenomena
are related to a promotion of the body's own natural immune response
systems. These compounds injected i.v. are acutely toxic, but the same
is not true if they are injected i.p. The toxicity is absent if the carbox-
ymethyl derivatives of mannans are used.

B. ALGINATES

Agar, algin, and *carrageenan* are important alginates. Agar and
carageenan are produced from the red algae and algin from the brown
algae. Most of the world's production of algin comes either from the
United States or the United Kingdom, with the United States supply-
ing 2×10^6 lb/year. Algin is derived from the cell walls of the brown
algae and is a linear glycuronan made up of β-D-mannuronic acid and
α-L-guluronic acid in a (1→4) linkage.

[β-D-mannuronic(1→4)]$_5$α-L-guluronic(1→4)β-D-mannuronic(1→4)[α-L-guluronic(1→4)]$_3$

A 3:2 ratio of mannuronic to guluronic acid residues is frequently
observed in the brown algaes. It is generally believed to be nontoxic
when administered orally but is, however, very toxic given i.v. There
may be some depression of weight gain when algin is fed at relatively
high levels (>10% of the diet). There is virtually no digestion or absorption of algin as determined by tracer studies.

Agar may be partially digestible. In both rats and guinea pigs, at
least, agar can be partially utilized as a nutrient. Agar is actually
composed of two components: agarose and agaropectin. Agarose is an
alternating chain of D-galactose and 3,6-anhydro-L-galactose with side
chains of 6-methyl-D-galactose. This compound has become especially
useful as a molecular sieve for the separation of proteins of various
molecular weights. Agaropectin contains, in addition to the components in agarose, sulfate esters and D-glucuronic acid. Agarose has the
better gelling characteristics of the two.

Carrageenan (food grade) appears not be utilized by animals. Alginates serve an important role as stabilizers and emulsifiers in foods. They are also used as edible coatings for meat to extend shelf life. Carrageenan is usually extracted from red algae, Irish moss, and is a 250,000 MW linear sulfated galactan. It occurs naturally in two forms: λ and κ. Other forms have also been described. The λ form is D-galactose 35% esterified with sulfate. The κ form also contains 3,6-anhydro-D-galactose in a 1:1.4 ratio with D-galactose. κ-Carageenan, which is 25% esterified with sulfate, is the form most capable of making a gel. It is used to increase viscosity in a number of products from foods to pharmaceuticals. It interacts readily with casein making it especially useful in dairy products. The λ component can be selectively extracted from the algae by soaking the plants in hot potassium, ammonium, or magnesium hydroxide. Other hydroxides of cations have also been employed. Selective extraction has been successfully applied to separation of the κ and λ from carrageenan extracts as well.

Food grade carrageenan, which has high molecular weight (100,000–500,000), has been reported to exert some physiological effects even though it is neither degraded nor absorbed following ingestion. Among these effects are antipeptic and antilipemic activities, decreased gastric secretion, and increased gut water content. These are all seen at high levels of carrageenan feeding but are not observed when carrageenan is added at the levels usually found in food. The antipeptic effect is probably due to an interaction of carageenan and the protein substrate and not to an alteration of the enzyme activity itself. Since a gum–substrate interaction is involved, relatively high amounts of carrageenan would be needed to interfere with utilization of dietary protein. The antilipemic effect of carageenan may well be similar to that of other nonabsorbable carbohydrates in that it may prevent cholesterol reabsorption in the form of bile acids.

Carrageenan has also been used medicinally in a degraded (20,000 MW) form. This type does not have any utility as a food stabilizer and has quite different physical properties. This form can be partly degraded and absorbed but still only to a very small extent. Degraded carrageenan has been used in Europe in the treatment of peptic ulcers. Presumably, it binds to the mucin of the stomach walls, providing an additional protective surface layer over the stomach.

C. PECTINS

Pectins are polymers of galacturonic acid with a variable number of carboxyl groups esterified with methyl groups. Pectin is not one substance but rather a group of substances with similar structures. Pectins are generally divided into two groups: low methyl ester pectins (3–5% methoxyl content) and high methyl ester pectins (7–8% methoxyl content). The pectins are particularly useful in jams and jellies and as stabilizers and thickeners in a variety of products such as dressings and frozen desserts. Pectin is often commercially obtained from citrus peel. In the making of jams and jellies, however, there is frequently enough natural pectin in the fruit to eliminate the necessity for exogenous pectin in order to achieve gelling. Apples, particularly, have a high pectin content (1.6% wet weight basis).

Pectin has found considerable utility in pharmaceutical applications. It is especially good in the treatment of diarrhea and has been used as a home remedy for this purpose for a very long time. The upper gastrointestinal tract of mammals is lacking in the ability to degrade pectin. The microorganisms in the colon, however, readily cause pectin decomposition to CO_2, acetate, and formate. It has been claimed that pectin has a slight bactericidal action, accounting for its antidiarrheal properties but this remains to be proved.

In a number of species, including humans, ingestion of pectin has been reported to increase the excretion of cholesterol but not always with concurrent decreases in total serum cholesterol. Pectin has been proposed to act by decreasing cholesterol absorption, altering intestinal microflora populations, or inhibiting bile acid reabsorption.

D. MICROBIAL POLYSACCHARIDES

Xanthan gum is the most commercially important of the microbially produced gums. Synthesis of this extracellular polysaccharide probably occurs inside the cell, then the completed chains are translocated through the cytoplasmic membrane to the cell surface. Culture conditions determine to what extent polysaccharides are produced. Maximum yield occurs under very aerobic conditions, and the product formed is not dependent on the carbon or energy source. A number of processes exist to separate the gum from the microorganisms and culture medium.

Xanthan gum is produced by the bacteria *Xanthomonas campestris*. It is a branched-chain polymer of glucose, mannose, and glucuronic acid with acetyl and pyruvic acid esters. It is a high molecular weight polymer (10^7 MW) and has a rod type conformation. It has a number of uses including stabilization of toothpaste, calf milk substitutes, and canned gravy type foods. Since the polymer is stable to salts and pH extremes, it is very useful under the corrosive conditions found in oil drilling.

Feeding studies have indicated that xanthan gum taken orally is nontoxic. At very high feeding levels, diarrhea may occur as often happens with many carbohydrates because of their osmotic properties. Xanthan gum may be partially broken down in the digestive tract (15% by tracer analysis) as the result of microbial action in the colon.

Dextran, another useful microbial exopolysaccharide, is obtained from *Leuconostoc mesenteroides*. It is 95% α-D$(1\rightarrow6)$-glucose, and the very long branches are all via the $\alpha(1\rightarrow3)$ linkages. Its main medical use is as a blood expander. Derivatives of dextrans are important as anticoagulants, antilipemics, and antiulcer agents. Dextran is also employed as a chromatographic material for protein purification and as an industrial gel.

A number of other microbial gums have been produced such as *curdlan* and *pullulan*. These gums have not yet been put to wide use but have various properties which give them good potential for many applications. There are increasing numbers of industrial situations both in food and nonfood industries where gums obtained from plant and nonplant sources may find application. Increasing efforts are being devoted to the development of suitable gums.

E. SUMMARY

Very high molecular weight polymers of glycosidically linked monosaccharides are capable of forming viscous gels when hydrated. These polymers are known as gums. Gums are obtained from intra- or extracellular sites of plants or microbes and fall into several categories: (1) mannans, galactomannans, and glucomannans; (2) alginates; (3) pectins; (4) microbial gums; and (5) others. Each may have special properties which make it useful for a particular application. They are used as thickeners, stabilizers, film formers, coagulants, colloids, and lubricants. Much of their utility is in industrial processes such as for oil drilling, improving the properties of food, and formulating pharmaceuticals. New potential uses develop every day for which gums are necessary if ones can be found with the appropriate properties.

REVIEW QUESTIONS

1. What are the sources of gums?
2. What are the basic physical properties of a gum?
3. What are the alginates?

BIBLIOGRAPHY

Lawrence, A. 1976. Natural Gums for Edible Purposes. Noyes Data Corp., Park Ridge, New Jersey.

Sandford, P. 1979. Exocellular, microbial polysaccharides. Adv. Carbohydr. Chem. Biochem. *36*, 265–313.

Southgate, D. 1976. Determination of Food Carbohydrates. Applied Science Publ., London.

Index